ELH DIET

PERMANENT WEIGHT LOSS
WITH
A HEALTHY DIET PLAN

ROBERT LALONDE

CLEAR PATH PUBLISHING

CANADA

Robert Lalonde/Clear Path Publishing
http://easyleanandhealthy.com/contact/

ELH DIET / Robert Lalonde. —1st ed.
ISBN 978-0-9940754-0-6

CONTENTS

Dedicated to All Dieters

Life is very simple but we insist on making it complicated.

CONFUCIUS

Introduction

In early 2000 I was lean and healthy and felt like I was on top of the world. Things were going great at work and I had almost completed all the requirements for my AACI designation. There were fewer than 4,000 Real Estate Appraisers with this designation in Canada at the time and my financial future looked bright.

In spring, my back started acting up and I was getting pretty serious back pain. This wasn't new for me as I had suffered a severe back injury in late 1989. I had managed to get back to work after a prolonged recovery period and although I was still in pain, it was being managed and I was able to live a fairly normal life. Until this most recent episode that is.

By June, my condition had worsened to the point that I could no longer sit at my desk for 15 minutes without having to get up and go for a walk. It got so bad the office manager told me I might as well go home. Two weeks later, I was on sick leave.

It turned out I had an 18mm kidney stone and I was booked for a lithotripsy procedure to break it up. Months later I still wasn't getting better and because they couldn't find a physical cause, I was diagnosed as suffering from depression and put on medication. While it was true that I was depressed from the pain and not being able to work, the depression was made much worse by an underlying kidney problem which was finally resolved by surgery in 2006, some 6 years later.

By this time I had put on a fair amount of weight and I craved sweets like ice cream like never before. On top of the poor eating habits, I was physically inactive throughout this entire time.

The surgery had helped the pain a fair bit, but my health did not return as expected. In December 2010 we found out why. I had a fairly large cancerous tumor and I would need to undergo another surgery to remove the affected section of the colon. Later, as I was doing research for this book, I learned that sugar feeds cancer cells. If you have a cancer, you will likely crave sugar a lot more than you used to, just as I did.

Back in 2000 I was in pretty good shape. I weighed about 170 pounds and ate a very healthy diet. With the onset of illness however, I gradually started eating differently. By 2014 my weight had ballooned to 205 lbs and I looked flushed and swollen. When I hit 208 lbs I decided something had to change.

I had been trying to lose weight for some time by cutting portion sizes but that didn't seem to be making much of a difference. I went back and re-read all the diet books I had and I reviewed the latest research papers online every day. I found that a lot has changed in the past 20 years when it comes to nutrition and weight loss. Some of what we knew still applies, but much of it has been found to be incorrect.

I've always made an effort to eat a healthy diet. I read labels and I always bought the healthiest foods I could. I would do this even when I bought snack foods. When I bought crackers, I would buy the healthy, natural products.

When I bought chips, I bought the low salt and low fat variety. I ate frozen yogurt instead of ice cream. I followed a natural foods diet as much as I could.

Yet suddenly, I was overweight and suffering from visible inflammation.

Truth be told, it didn't really happen all that suddenly. Like many others, the treats I would enjoy on occasion slowly got out of hand. In the beginning, I would occasionally have a small bowl of frozen yogurt after dinner. Eventually, I started craving this more and more until I was having it every day. Then I started having a second serving the odd time. In the end, I just started using a larger bowl.

Like many people, I had more than one favorite treat. Besides the frozen yogurt, I also enjoyed the occasional cookie and the odd bowl of potato chips. Unfortunately, what happened with the frozen yogurt also happened with the cookies and potato chips.

The simple truth is this: whether it's loose change and small bills you stuff into a jar every day or extra calories you stuff into your body, it will add up over time.

I learned that while it's important to eat good natural food, not all foods affect us the same way. A calorie is not a calorie once it enters our body.

Different foods affect us in different ways and some foods lead to more weight gain than others.

Once you understand this, you can take advantage of the situation and combine some foods with others to avoid gaining weight. I learned that it's not necessary to eat smaller portions or eat less often to lose weight or to maintain body weight once the extra pounds have been shed.

By using this approach, I lost 38 lbs in about 6 months and I now weigh what I did back in 2000. I did this without eating less food or taking up an exercise program.

If you're looking for a sensible way to lose weight permanently with a healthy diet plan, you're in the right place. The ELH DIET will lead you through all the steps to trim the excess weight off and it will show you how to stop craving the foods that provide empty calories and lead you to gain weight. You get to eat lots of food and you will gain control over your weight in a way that makes it easy to keep the weight off for good.

About The Author

Robert Lalonde is a recent cancer survivor. He lives in the Georgian Bay area in Ontario, Canada with his wife Marianne and their Shi Tzu, Lucy.

Robert studied Real Estate Appraisal in college and Real Property Assessment through UBC. He worked as a Commercial Property Tax Consultant in Toronto, Canada, representing owners of hotels, office buildings and shopping malls before various tribunals for tax appeals.

From The Author

I'm not overly fond of the term Paleo diet, but that seems to be the popular name for diets that recommend eating the good wholesome foods we grew up on before all the mass produced foods hit the shelves.

The early Paleo diets were overly restrictive based on poor information. Legumes, for example were not allowed, because the early adopters were misinformed as to whether or not our ancestors ate legumes. It turns out some of them did.

The most important questions to ask when considering whether or not to eat a food are: "is it a natural food and how does it impact our health?"

This book is the result of research I carried out to lose weight and regain my health after a battle with cancer. I've read many books and reviewed countless studies by specialists to gain a better understanding about dieting and how different foods affect our health.

In this book, I cut through all the hype and marketing we are subjected to every day to find an answer to these two questions:

1. What is the best way to lose weight and keep it off?

2. Does the food we eat contribute to chronic illnesses?

We Are What We Eat

Our lifestyle and environmental factors expose us to chemical tags that change our DNA. In other words, our DNA can change not only from bad habits like smoking, but also because of what we eat and drink, the medicines we take and the pollutants we get exposed to on a daily basis.

Some of these changes to our DNA are harmless but *others trigger disease or increase the severity of the illness.* Changes to DNA have been linked to various cancers, diabetes, autoimmune diseases and even mental illness.

> ***As I delved deeper into the causes and cures of cancer, I realized that diet, obesity and cancer are all linked together.***

We may not be able to control what it is we eat as much as we like, but we can become informed consumers and we must take some control and responsibility for our own health and well-being. No one else is going to do this for us.

We also need to develop a better understanding of how our body reacts to the foods we eat. Not all calories are the same once they enter our body and we can use tools like the glycemic index and the glycemic load to minimize insulin spikes and weight gain.

We lead busy lives and we're often tempted to use prepared foods to free up a bit of extra time. Working mothers look for convenience foods and single people eat in fast food restaurants. Pizza and takeout food is a quick fix as we try to find a bit of time to relax from the tedium of making meals.

THE WEIGHT CONNECTION

Most of us don't worry about getting cancer – I sure didn't. But do you worry about your weight? Most people are concerned about how they look but they're not as aware as they should be about the direct connection between weight and chronic illness. *I was overweight for a number of years before my cancer was discovered and it is estimated that one out of three cancers are directly related to diet.*

More than two thirds of the people in developed countries around the world are either overweight or obese. And obesity is associated with increased risk for cancers of the esophagus, breast, colon, kidney, pancreas and a host of others.

Obese people are also at higher risk for coronary heart disease, stroke, high blood pressure and diabetes. *The food we eat and the physical activity we engage in is where we can take charge and reduce our risk to develop all these conditions.*

It's never too late to make improvements. If you've already suffered a critical illness as I have, a better diet isn't going to turn back the clock, but it will improve your health and well-being.

It is my hope that I can convince you to make a few changes in your life; changes that will improve your quality of life and hopefully keep you healthier and prevent illness that could be avoided.

CHAPTER 1

Is Long Term Weight Loss Possible

Is it possible for a person who is overweight or obese to lose weight and keep it off? The answer is a definite yes. There is a way to lose weight and keep it off long term.

A missing piece of the puzzle with most diets is that they do not address the food cravings and the constant hunger signals that are behind the weight control problems experienced by many people. You need a diet that stops you from craving foods you shouldn't be eating in the first place.

Moderation Wins The Day

Many diet plans offer up some good advice. Where most fall short is in having too narrow a focus. We are complex beings with a number of interconnected systems, each of which has an effect on the entire organism.

Diets advocating that you should cut out an entire food group, as in a no-carb or very low carb diet, are likely to cause problems in the long run. Besides, there is no proof that eating carbohydrates in moderation is likely to cause problems unless you are intolerant or allergic to some of the foods in this category.

As for the argument that carbohydrates are not the most nutritionally dense foods, most of us, excepting elite athletes, don't view food simply as fuel. It is that, but it's so much more!

If you want to lose weight and stop craving bad food this is the book for you.

Working With Your Metabolism

One of our survival skills as a species is the ability to store excess food in the form of fat. We have evolved this way so we can use the stored fat as a source of energy when food becomes scarce.

However, because food is always available at the nearest grocer or convenience store in modern times, this fat storage mechanism has become a curse for many people.

A diet that has you cut back on food portions will trigger this mechanism and set you up for rebound weight gain down the road.

The ELH DIET is a healthy diet plan that will lead you through the steps to lose weight in a way that won't set you up for failure a few months down the road

A Healthy Diet Plan

It is difficult to lose weight if you eat a lot of processed foods. Processed foods are often loaded with added sugar or worse, High Fructose Corn Syrup. Eating too much sugar has devastating effects on your metabolism that go way beyond calorie content.

These foods make your body release too much insulin which causes your blood sugar level to shoot up and then drop below where it was before you ate. Lower blood sugar levels make you crave sugary foods, starting the cycle anew and leaving you stuck in a never ending loop.

Letting Old Habits Go

We act out of habit to a large extent and we need to change these habits if we want to lose weight. Fortunately, we can do this fairly quickly with the right plan and the will to make a change.

No change will take place unless you make a firm decision to change and then act on that decision.

The ELH DIET plan works – all you have to do is follow the program.

The recommendations for the Standard North American Diet (SAD) are that we should eat mostly carbohydrates. A high carbohydrate intake is still being recommended today, even though one third of the population is obese!

Physicians who treat obese patients then place these people on a carbohydrate restricted diet so they can lose weight. It's no wonder people are confused and don't know what to eat!

What Goes In Matters

It's important to have a basic understanding of our lymphatic system because it is our drainage system. It might help you decide why it matters whether you eat processed and genetically modified foods.

Your body will try to get rid of anything it considers foreign matter. Chemicals and foods that are not found in nature certainly fall into this category. You will see your skin clear up quickly and dramatically if you just cut back on these foods, let alone eliminate them entirely from your diet!

This book can change your life. It will show you how to lose weight and how to keep it off.

Some of the food we eat causes low level inflammation and this sets us up for a number of health problems. You will learn to read your body in the first two stages of this diet and you will become aware of any food sensitivity you might have.

This will allow you to make further changes to your diet that will improve your health beyond just losing weight.

There is absolutely nothing to count and you can have as much real food as you want. You will learn that it's not only about what you eat; it's also about how eating certain foods leads your body to store fat for a rainy day that just isn't coming.

CHAPTER 2

OBESITY AND ITS CAUSES

Obesity is recognized as a chronic disease and it is the second leading cause of preventable death after smoking. Rates of obesity have been on the rise and obesity is now considered a major health risk.

Approximately one-third of adults are considered to be obese. That number doubles to two-thirds when you include people who are overweight and possibly pre-diabetic.

The percentage of individuals who are simply overweight has been fairly steady at about 30 percent. However, the rate of obesity has been increasing rapidly in the past 30 years as shown in this chart:

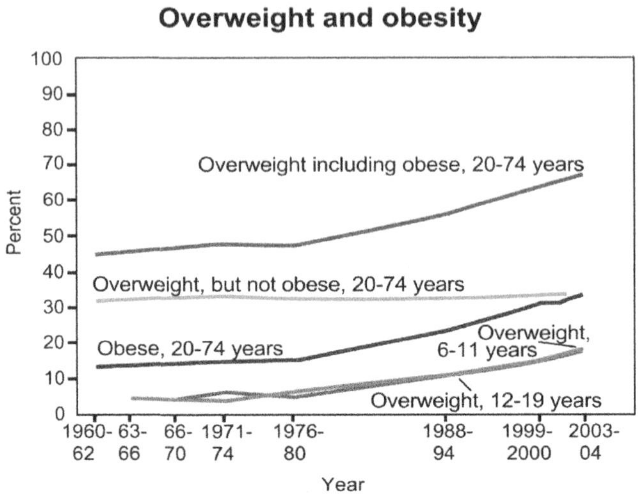

SOURCES: Centers for Disease Control and Prevention, National Center for Health Statistics, *Health, United States. 2006*, Figure 13. Data from National Health and Nutrition Examination Survey

---

Increased Calorie Intake

It is a fact that we are consuming about 30 percent more calories in America today than we were 40 years ago. This is the basis of the *eat less, do more* weight loss plans.

However, the idea that eating too much and exercising too little is the cause of obesity is an oversimplification and it is not very helpful to people who need a simple and practical way to lose weight.

Increased Consumption of Prepared Food

I've tried cutting portion size in an effort to lose weight, as have many others. It didn't work for me and it doesn't work for most people and I'll explain why later.

What is useful is an understanding of where those extra calories come from. This chart was created using data from the USDA Economic Research Service, Loss-Adjusted Food Availability:

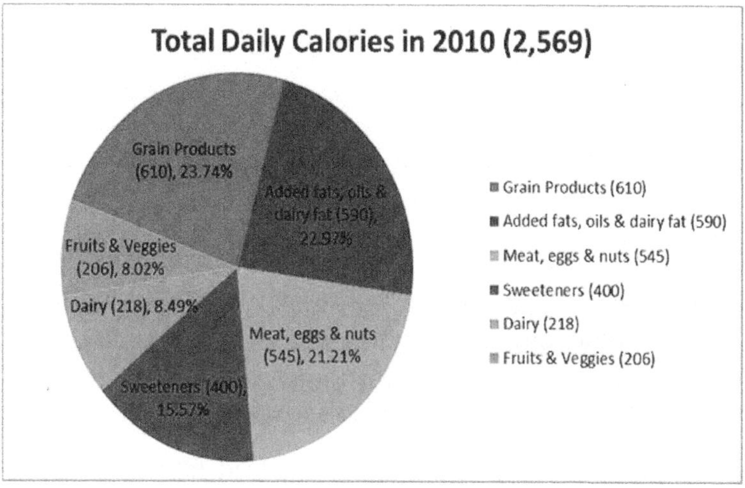

The *Added fats, oils & dairy fat category* and the *Sweeteners category*, both refer to items that are added during processing or preparation of foods. Together, they make up 38.54 percent of the daily calorie intake of the average American.

By cutting back or eliminating processed and prepared foods you can easily reduce your calorie intake by 20 percent.

Body Fat Baseline Levels

Researchers have discovered that we have a network of circuits in the brain that have the job of maintaining our current amount of body fat. This is done by regulating our food intake, our energy expenditure and the storage of energy in our fat tissue.

LEPTIN – WHY YOU'RE STILL HUNGRY.

One of the more interesting bits of new information in recent years was the discovery of the hormone leptin. It turns out that our fat tissue produces this hormone and uses it to communicate with the brain.

As we lose fat by dieting, our reduced fat mass signals the brain to stimulate hunger and to use calories more efficiently so we can regain the body fat we just lost! The exact opposite happens if you eat too much and put on weight. The increase in fat mass produces leptin and signals the brain to suppress your appetite and use up more calories until body fat goes back to normal.[1]

Leptin and a few other hormones are part of a negative feedback loop that acts to keep your fat mass in a specific range much like a thermostat does for the temperature in your home.

When this system stops working properly or starts to defend fat stores more than it should, we gain weight. It's also why it's so hard to keep weight off when you diet.

Even though you still have too much fat, your brain thinks it needs to recapture what was lost![2]

Cortisol and Stress

Cortisol is a steroid hormone that regulates energy. In our ever-stressed, fast-paced lifestyle, our bodies are pumping out cortisol almost constantly. Elevated cortisol over the long term consistently produces glucose and leads to increased blood sugar levels and weight gain. It can also increase your appetite and cravings for high-calorie foods.

Causes of Obesity That You Can Control

There are many factors that contribute to obesity. If you make small adjustments in each of these categories, the cumulative effect will be quite noticeable.

Here are 10 factors that you can minimize to help you lose weight:

1. Refined carbohydrates

Refined carbs drive insulin and insulin drives fat deposition. So when it comes to accumulating fat, refined carbs are bad calories because they boost insulin and increase fat storage.

2. Junk Food

When rats were fed a diet of junk food, they ignored their regular food and gained a lot of fat quickly. It turns out that junk food happens to be the most effective way to overwhelm the body's fat balancing system. What's worse is, rats and humans eventually become highly motivated to obtain junk food. In experiments, the rats would endure cold temperatures and even electric shock to get at junk food, even when their regular food was sitting right there![3]

3. Too Many Carbohydrates

There are many studies that confirm a low-glycemic load diet can help with weight loss, with one exception, the 'Omni carb trial.[4]

However, this trial looked at the effectiveness of high vs a low glycemic index diets in various studies. This strikes me as odd, because the glycemic index relates to individual foods consumed in isolation from other foods. Once you start eating foods in combination, the glycemic index no longer applies, and perhaps that's why they found it wasn't useful.

The study did show one item of importance though, and that is:

All high carbohydrate diets increased insulin sensitivity by 20 percent in a 5 week period.

4. Processed Foods

Most foods we eat are processed in some way. But there's a difference between mechanical processing and chemical processing.

Mass produced foods that have been chemically processed and are made with refined ingredients and artificial substances are generally known as processed foods.

Processed foods are usually loaded with sugar or High Fructose Corn Syrup. Many of these products have been engineered to be incredibly rewarding to the brain and intentionally cause over consumption.

These foods are high in refined carbs and low in fiber which creates greater insulin spikes that drive the body to store fat. Unhealthy fats used in processing also cause inflammation which increases the risk of heart disease.

5. Salt

Salt affects weight gain in three ways. First, a higher salt intake makes your body retain more water. Second, salty foods increase thirst, and many people quench that thirst with beverages that are packed with calories. Third, salt enhances the taste of foods and may encourage overeating. Bland foods rarely encourage overeating.

About 70 percent of the sodium in the American diet comes from processed foods. This is another compelling reason to stop eating processed foods.

6. Toxic Load

As your liver becomes overburdened with toxins, it causes imbalances that can lead to weight gain. These imbalances include blood sugar imbalance, essential fatty acid deficiency and slowed metabolism.

A high toxic load also causes a stagnant lymph flow. Your body holds toxins and body weight accumulates.

7. Sugar

One of the major causes of our expanding waistlines and rapidly deteriorating health is sugar and artificial sugar substitutes.

The more sugar in the blood stream, the more insulin is released. Insulin helps store all of this glucose in the liver and muscles as glycogen, and in fat cells as triglycerides.[5]

Note: There are different kinds of sugar. Anything that ends with 'ose' is a sugar.

8. Dieting

Your body experiences the dieting process as a form of starvation. Your cells don't know that you're voluntarily restricting your food intake so your body shifts into famine survival mode causing your metabolism to slow down and food cravings to escalate.

This effect compounds with each diet as your body adapts and learns to function on fewer calories. This is the underlying mechanism that causes people to gain weight as they come off each diet.

9. Eating Diet Foods

Most so-called diet drinks and diet foods use one or more artificial sweeteners to replace sugar. Unfortunately for dieters, the artificial sweeteners cause 50 percent more weight gain than drinks sweetened with regular sugar.[6]

10. Lack of exercise

We all know that a lack of exercise affects our weight. It is estimated that a quarter of the population is completely sedentary while up to 55 percent are not getting enough exercise to promote good health.

Without enough exercise, your metabolism slows down, your lymph system becomes congested and your lean muscle mass becomes depleted. All these factors facilitate weight gain.

What About Fats

I used to eat very little fat. In fact, I used to trim all the fat off any meat I ate, *yet I was overweight.*

Over the past 30 years, most people have cut their fat intake by 30 percent and yet more of us are fat today than ever before. If dietary fat was really the problem, we'd all be thin and healthy by now. But we're not!

In the years we've been trimming fat from our diets, type II diabetes has tripled and obesity has skyrocketed. What did we replace the fat calories with in our diet? *Refined carbohydrates.*

The truth has finally come out: fat was never the problem.

The fat content in a meal is part of what makes you feel full and satiated. Eating good fats and avoiding bad fats is part of a good diet. Studies show fat was never the problem.[7]

For example, Omega-3 fats help you burn fat by helping your body respond to leptin. *Since it's leptin that signals the brain to tell your body to suppress your appetite, eating fats can actually make you eat less and lose weight.*

It's important to note that it's not carbohydrates from healthy foods that have caused the problem.

NOTES

[1] Reviews in Undergraduate Research, Vol. 2, 12-18 , 2003 "Leptin As Fat Orchestrator" Jaime Hennessey1, Communicated by: Dr. Andrew Dobson

[2] The Journal of Clinical Endocrinology and Metabolism "Clinical review: Regulation of food intake, energy balance, and body fat mass: implications for the pathogenesis and treatment of obesity" Guyenet SJ, Schwartz MW (http://www.ncbi.nlm.nih.gov/pmc/articles/PMC3319208)

[3] USNC Dietary obesity in adult rats: similarities to hypotha-lamic and human obesity syndromes Sclafani A, SpringerD.
(http://www.ncbi.nlm.nih.gov/pubmed/1013192)

[4] USNC - Sacks FM, et al. "Effects of High vs Low Glycemic Index of Dietary Carbohydrate on Cardiovascular Disease Risk Factors and Insulin Sensitivity. The OmniCarb Randomized Clinical Trial
(http://www.ncbi.nlm.nih.gov/pubmed/25514303

[5] Erya E. Mehran et al. "Hyperinsulinemia Drives Diet-Induced Obesity Independently of Brain Insulin Production"
(http://www.sciencedirect.com/science/article/pii/S1550413112004536)

[6] Harvard School of Public Medicine "Artificial Sweeteners" (http://www.hsph.harvard.edu/nutritionsource/healthy-drinks/artificial-sweeteners/)

[7] AJCN "Meta-analysis of prospective cohort studies evaluating the association of saturated fat with cardiovascular disease" Patty W. Siri et al. (http://ajcn.nutrition.org/content/early/2010/01/13/ajcn.2009.27725.abstract)

CHAPTER 3

Foods and Insulin

The hormone insulin is needed for glucose to enter our cells and be used for energy.

As the glucose level in your bloodstream rises after you eat, your pancreas secretes insulin which allows glucose to enter the cells. The level of glucose in the bloodstream then returns to its pre-meal level.

Glucose is either used by your cells for your immediate energy needs or it is stored for an energy reserve as glycogen in the cells of the liver and muscles or as triglycerides in your fatty tissues.

Within two hours after a meal we begin storing any excess glucose.

Diabetes and Pre-Diabetes

I was considered pre-diabetic before I went on this diet. These are the early stages of the disease, and it was a wake-up call when my doctor gave me the news.

Diabetes is basically a disease of glucose intolerance. High blood glucose is the cause and *the best diet to control diabetes or pre-diabetes is a low-carbohydrate diet.* By limiting our intake to low glycemic load carbs, our blood glucose levels will drop more quickly and so will body fat.

Hypoglycemia

In a healthy person, insulin secretion is correctly balanced with the amount of glucose entering the bloodstream. In some people however, the secretion of insulin is excessive. This results in an abnormally rapid drop in the blood glucose (blood sugar) level after a meal if the pancreas overshoots on insulin production.

The result is too little glucose in the blood. This condition is called reactive hypoglycemia and it occurs in people who do not have diabetes.

The person experiencing this may become weak, irritable, dizzy or develop a headache. They will probably also become very hungry within an hour or two after a meal and crave sugar or starchy foods. Another dose of carbohydrates starts the cycle over again.[1]

As a result, your appetite is out of balance with your body's actual need for food, and the glucose that is being driven out of the bloodstream and into the cells gets stored as fat.

A high level of insulin also activates an enzyme called lipoprotein lipase. This enzyme increases the production of triglycerides from any fatty acids you eat in a meal.

Excess insulin promotes the storage of any fat you eat.

Burning Fat

I used to eat way too many high glycemic carbohydrates like rice and potatoes and that's why I couldn't lose weight even when I cut down portion size and ate less food. High glycemic carbs spike our insulin and excess carbs and dietary fat are more likely to be stored as fat.

To make things worse, those high insulin levels obstruct the activity of the enzyme triglyceride lipase that breaks down stored fat for use as energy.

If you have chronically high insulin, you cannot burn your own body fat! [2]

If a person continually over-produces insulin a state of insulin resistance results and insulin becomes less effective at getting glucose into the cells to be used for energy or stored for future use. Since blood sugar levels don't drop as quickly after a meal in a person with insulin resistance, the pancreas keeps secreting more insulin which becomes less and less effective in doing its job.

Insulin resistance is a pre-diabetic state. It can result in weight gain and other symptoms which characterize metabolic syndrome such as high blood pressure and abnormal blood fat levels. Ironically, *fasting or skipping meals can also cause insulin resistance, possibly by increasing cortisol levels.*[3]

NOTES

[1] Medline Plus "Hypoglycemia" (http://www.nlm.nih.gov/medlineplus/hypoglycemia.html)

[2] Diabetes Health "Why Eating Too Many Carbs Makes You Fat" Barry Groves (http://diabeteshealth.com/read/2007/04/24/5143/why-eating-too-many-carbs-makes-you-fat/)

[3] Today's Dietician "Cortisol — Its Role in Stress, Inflammation, and Indications for Diet Therapy Dina Aronson (http://www.todaysdietitian.com/newarchives/111609p38.shtml)

CHAPTER 4

Ketosis – Burning Fat

Your body stores fat reserves that can be converted into usable energy at times when food isn't available.

The bear is the classic example used to demonstrate this. During the long winter months, the bear utilizes his fat storage to maintain his bodily functions. The bear is in a state called ketosis.

What we call fat, scientists call triglycerides. Fat, or triglycerides, consists of one molecule of glycerol and three molecules of long-chain fatty acid.

When you break down fat, you release glycerol and fatty acids. *Glycerol is then converted into glucose in the liver and is used as energy.* Fatty acids break down into Acetyl-Co A by a process call beta oxidation. Acetyl-Co A can enter into the mitochondria of the cell and go through the Krebs Cycle and produce energy. During this process, by-products called ketone bodies are formed.[1]

Ketogenic Diets

Carb reduced diets are meant to shift our metabolism from using glucose to using fat, so they fall in the ketogenic diet category.

People who want to switch to burning fat all day long restrict their carb intake to 100 grams a day or less to induce certain adaptations.

I don't worry about the exact amount of carbs I eat and I don't think it's necessary for you to worry about it either. As long as you cut down on your high glycemic load carb intake, you will lose weight.

Fuel Metabolism on a Ketogenic Diet

In a normal diet your body runs on a mix of carbs, protein and fat. When you remove carbs from your diet, the body's supplies are quickly depleted and your body has to find an alternative fuel for energy. One of these fuels is free fatty acids (FFA). However, some parts of the body like the brain and nervous system are unable to use FFA for fuel, but they can use ketone bodies.

Ketone bodies are a by-product of the incomplete breakdown of FFA in the liver. They are a fat-derived fuel for tissues like the brain.

As the production of ketone bodies accelerates, they accumulate in the bloodstream and cause a metabolic state called ketosis. At the same time, there's a decrease in the use of glucose and protein for energy

Ketogenic diets are perfectly suited for people who want to maintain lean body mass while they lose fat.

HORMONES AND THE KETOGENIC DIET

When you cut or remove carbs from your diet, your insulin levels go down and your glucagon levels go up. This causes an increase in FFA being released from fat cells and increases FFA burning in the liver.

The accelerated FFA burning in the liver leads to the production of ketones and the state of ketosis.

THE BASICS OF FUEL UTILIZATION

In The Ketogenic Diet Lyle MacDonald says our body uses four primary fuels: glucose, protein, free fatty acids, and ketones. These fuels are stored in varying proportions in your body.[2]

The primary form of stored fuel is triglycerides (fat) which are stored in the fatty tissue. Glucose and protein make up secondary sources. These fuels are used in varying proportions depending on the metabolic state of the body.

The main determinant of which fuel gets used is the amount of carbs in your diet.

In a typical diet, ketones play a non-existent role in energy production. In fasting or a ketogenic diet, ketones play a larger role in energy production, especially in the brain.

The information in this chart comes from the "Textbook of Biochemistry with Clinical Correlations 4th ed." Ed. Thomas M. Devlin. Wiley-Liss. As you can see in the chart, carb stores are minimal in comparison to protein and fat and are only sufficient to sustain the body for about one day.

Comparison of bodily fuels in a 150 lb man with 22% body fat		
Tissue	Average weight (lbs)	Caloric worth (kcal)
Adipose tissue triglyceride	33	135,000
Muscle protein	13	24,000
Carbohydrate stores (3 categories)		
Muscle glycogen (normal)	0.25	480
Liver glycogen	0.5	280
Blood glucose	0.04	80
Total carbohydrate stores	**0.8**	**840**

Relationships in Fuel Use

Typically, the body will use a given fuel in proportion to its concentration in the bloodstream. So if glucose increases in the bloodstream, the body will utilize that fuel in preference to others. By the same token, if the concentrations of a given fuel decrease in the bloodstream, the body will use less of that fuel.

When you decrease your carb intake, your body shifts to using fat as its primary fuel.

GLUCOSE AND PROTEIN USE

The preferred fuel for most tissues in the body is glucose, with the exception of the heart, which uses a mix of glucose, FFA and ketones.

The major source of glucose in the body is from dietary carbs. However, through a process called gluconeogenesis, other substances can be converted to glucose in the liver and kidney. This includes certain amino acids, especially alanine and glutamine.

There is little gluconeogenesis from the body's protein stores when there are normal amounts of glucose. This has led many to state that carbs have a protein sparing effect in that they prevent the breakdown of protein to make glucose. This same high carb intake also decreases the use of fat for fuel.

In addition to being protein sparing, carbs are also fat sparing

It is important to have an adequate protein intake during the first few weeks of a ketogenic diet to prevent muscle loss. Without enough protein in your diet, body protein will be scavenged for gluconeogenesis.

FREE FATTY ACIDS (FFA) AND KETONES

Most tissues of the body, including skeletal muscle, the heart, and most organs, can use FFA for fuel if it is available. However, there are other tissues such as the brain, red blood cells, the renal medulla, bone marrow and Type II muscle fibers which cannot use FFA and require glucose.

The fact that the brain is incapable of using FFA for fuel has led to the misconceptions that the brain can only use glucose for fuel. While it is true that the brain normally runs on glucose, the brain will use ketones for fuel if they are available.

The brain can actually draw up to 75 percent of its total energy requirements from ketones after adaptation. As with glucose and FFA, the use of ketones is related to their availability.

Typically, ketone concentrations are so low that they provide a negligible amount of energy to the tissues. As ketone concentrations increase, most tissues in the body begin to derive some portion of their energy from ketones. The liver is an exception as it relies on FFA.

After three weeks, most tissues will meet their energy requirements almost exclusively through the breakdown of FFA. This is thought to be an adaptation to ensure adequate ketone levels for the brain.

Except in the case of Type I diabetes, ketones will only be present in the bloodstream under conditions where FFA use by the body has increased. Generally, it is assumed that a large increase in FFA use is accompanied by an increase in ketone utilization.

RELATIONSHIP BETWEEN CARBS AND FAT

As long as muscle and liver glycogen stores are not completely filled, the body is able to store or burn off excess dietary carbohydrates.

This occurs at the expense of fat burning, meaning most dietary fat ingested in a high carb diet gets stored as fat.

The perfect storm in terms of fat gain is consuming a diet that is high-carb AND high-fat, combined with an inactive lifestyle.

When glycogen stores are chronically overfilled and you consume a large amount of carbohydrates, fat burning is almost completely blocked and any dietary fat consumed is stored.

This led to the idea of limiting dietary fat for weight loss. But we now know that eating more carbs is what creates fat. And, since dietary fat is what makes you feel full, limiting dietary fats is not the best strategy - and we have history to prove that!

The ketogenic diet approaches this problem from the opposite direction. Reducing your carb intake helps control hunger and improves fat metabolism which leads to reduced body weight.[3]

The more you reduce your carb intake, the easier it is to burn fat.

NOTES

[1]Wikipedia "ketosis"

(http://en.wikipedia.org/wiki/Ketosis)

[2]The ketogenic diet: a complete guide for dieters and practitioners By: McDonald, Lyle.
Morris Pub. 1998

[3] PMC "Ketogenic Diet for Obesity: Friend or Foe?" Antonio
Paoli (http://www.ncbi.nlm.nih.gov/pmc/articles/PMC3945587/)

CHAPTER 5

Do You Need Carbohydrates

It *is* true that you can live without carbs, and there are actually a few diets that are based on zero or near zero carb intake.

I could understand someone taking this approach if we knew that all carbs were bad, but that's not the case!

> *Many carbohydrates are good for you and they provide healthy micro-nutrients.*

Carbohydrates often get a bad rap especially when it comes to weight gain. But not all carbs are bad. They have numerous health benefits and they are necessary as you become more active. They also provide a low cost source of energy for many people who live on limited budgets.

UNDERSTANDING CARBOHYDRATES

Carbohydrates are a type of macronutrient found naturally in many foods. Food manufacturers also add carbs to processed foods in the form of starch or added sugar.

Natural sources of carbs include fruits, vegetables, milk, nuts, grains, seeds and legumes.

Three Main Types of Carbohydrates

Three Main Types of Carbohydrates	
Sugar	The simplest form of carbs. Sugars include fruit sugar (fructose), table sugar (sucrose) and milk sugar (lactose).
Starch	A complex carb made of many sugar units bonded together. Occurs naturally in grains and cooked dry beans and peas.
Fiber	Another complex carb. Occurs naturally in fruits, vegetables, whole grains and cooked dry beans and peas.

HOW MANY CARBOHYDRATES ARE NEEDED?

There is NO right amount of carbohydrates to eat for everyone. What we do know is this: generally speaking, the more active your lifestyle, the more carbs you should eat.

It's important to understand how different lifestyles and health factors affect carb usage. You also need to factor in your own personal experience – we're not all the same.

IMPORTANT FACTORS TO CONSIDER ARE:

Current Health and Insulin Resistance

Insulin resistance can lead to hyperinsulinia, increased inflammation and an increased risk for all degenerative diseases.

Most overweight or obese people are already in a state of insulin resistance and they can reverse that by lowering their carb intake and eliminating all high GI and GL foods.

Current Activity Level

What should determine your carb intake is how often and how intensely you work out.

If walking is your main form of exercise, you're not going to use the same amount of muscle glycogen as someone who is active in sports or does serious weight training.

When it comes to carbs, eat for your activity level

If your goal is weight loss and you are overweight, not very active, and/or only do low intensity activity like walking – you need a lower carb approach to keep insulin low, reverse insulin resistance and slowly burn stored fat all day.

If you work at a desk job and are moderately active you can have a higher carb intake. Ideal weight loss will come from reducing your carb intake so you can burn fat most of the time.

CHAPTER 6

WHAT ABOUT FAT

There's a myth that refuses to die. It goes like this: *eating fat makes you fat.*[1]

If you just look at calories this would appear to make sense. After all, fat contains 9 calories per gram, while carbs and proteins contain 4 calories per gram. If calories were the only thing to consider, it would stand to reason that you would put on more weight if you were to eat fat rather than proteins or carbs.

But, it's not just about the number of calories you take in; it's also about how different foods affect your metabolism.

THE IMPORTANCE OF FAT IN THE DIET

Fat is an essential part of every single cell membrane in your body and it's important to us for a number of reasons.

Fat is required to properly digest and assimilate the fat-soluble vitamins A, D, E and K. That's why pasteurized skim milk fortified with synthetic vitamin D is a silly idea.

Nature provides the fat required to digest these vitamins in many foods. For example, the fat in egg yolks allows the body to access the vitamins A and D that are so plentiful in eggs.

Fats are also needed for the proper use of proteins. All the egg whites in the world won't do you any good if you're not eating them with the fats in the yolk that allow you to access that protein properly.

WHY YOU NEED GOOD FATS

- Fats are a source of consistent, smooth - burning energy.
- Fats also slow the absorption of food and make you feel full after a meal.
- Fats don't trigger the release of insulin and fat storage like carbs do.

Sugar and foods that convert to sugar quickly, like bread, pastas and cereal lead to overeating and binging because they don't satiate and because of the insulin reaction. After insulin does its job of storing that extra sugar as fat, guess what happens? Your blood sugar drops and you are back in low-blood sugar space. And guess what you'll crave then? **More sugar!**

That's the vicious cycle you need to break!

All Fats Are Not Created Equal

Industrially processed oils and rancid fats are everywhere in the modern diet. These are extremely harmful to your health *and* your waistline.[2]

Essential Fatty Acids

Essential fatty acids are fats that we need to sustain good health, *but can't produce on our own.*

There are two fatty acids needed by the human body: alpha-linolenic acid, and linoleic acid, commonly known as Omega-3 and Omega-6 fatty acids, respectively.

What Makes Them Essential

They're essential because our body can't produce them. Essential fatty acids are the good fats that are essential for the human body to function properly.

Omega fatty acids aid in the regulation of blood pressure, heart rate, and reproductive ability and trigger the body to fight off infection.

Having a deficiency in omega fatty acids has been found to play a role in various health conditions such as insulin resistance, heart attacks, strokes, obesity, lupus and Alzheimer's disease to name a few.

Omega-3 Fatty Acid (Alpha-Linolenic Acid)

Omega-3 is known as the heart healthy fat. Omega-3s are linked to improving blood circulation, flexibility of red blood cells, and formation of cellular walls. They are essential for proper intracellular activity.

Deficient Omega-3 levels have been linked to many health concerns and disorders such as high cholesterol, heart disease, blood clots, high blood pressure, lower immune function, poor vision, nerve sensation, and even diminishing mental capacities like memory loss. Omega-3s help reduce Alzheimers and dementia.

FOODS THAT CONTAIN OMEGA-3'S:

- Fish: Salmon, mackerel, sardines, anchovies and albacore tuna
- Oils: Krill oil, fish oil, flaxseed, hempseed, canola, soybean and wheat germ
- Seeds: Flaxseed, hempseed, pumpkin, sesame and flaxseed meal
- Nuts: Brazil and walnut
- Leafy Greens: Kale, spinach, purslane, mustard greens and collards

Krill oil has the highest level of Omega-3 of any other food and it's my preferred source. To receive the full benefits of Omega-3 fatty acids try to consume the food in a raw, unrefined state.

Omega-6 Fatty Acid (Linoleic)

Omega-6 fatty acids are involved in metabolic functions and the overall health of your nervous system. Consuming Omega-6 fatty acids can improve conditions like premenstrual syndrome, rheumatoid arthritis, skin disorders and diabetic neuropathy.

Omega-3 and Omega-6 fatty acids are primarily found in natural, unrefined foods.

Foods That Contain Omega 6 Fats

- Oils: Hempseed, flaxseed, grapeseed, olive, borage, evening primrose, black currant and chestnut
- Seeds: Flaxseed, hempseed, pumpkin and sunflower
- Nuts: Pine and pistachio
- Flaxseed Meal
- Chicken
- Olives

Heat destroys the beneficial acids in oils so you should always store your products in the refrigerator. Avoid processed and hydrogenated oils.

Corn, safflower, sunflower, cottonseed, and soybean oils also contain Omega-6 fatty acids, but it's difficult to find them unrefined or non-GMO.

Omega-9 Fatty Acids (Oleic) A Semi-Essential

While Omega-9 fatty acid is not essential, it is necessary.

Omega-9 fatty acids lower the risk of arteriosclerosis (hardening of the arteries) and heart attacks. You may find Omega-9 fatty acids in oils and nuts. The most common are olive and sesame oils, avocados, macadamia nuts, peanuts, pecans, almonds, pistachios, hazelnuts, and cashews.

Saturated Fats

Saturated fat intake does raise blood cholesterol levels *in the short term*, but not in long term use.[3] Like many people, I'm still having a hard time figuring out how to deal with this information.

We've been told for so long to avoid saturated fat it's going to take some time to understand how we should change our diet. Studies show there is some variation in how individuals respond to dietary saturated fat, but long-term studies show no net change in cholesterol levels.

Even those people who originally thought fat intake was associated with heart disease have ceased believing this for over 20 years.

Ancel Keys, who was largely credited as the founder of the idea that saturated fats caused heart disease wrote a letter to the New England Journal of Medicine in 1991 saying:

"Dietary cholesterol has an important effect on the cholesterol level in the blood of chickens and rabbits, but many controlled experiments have shown that dietary cholesterol has a limited effect in humans".

Adding cholesterol to a cholesterol-free diet raises the blood level in humans, but when added to an unrestricted diet, it has a minimal effect.

Fats Are Not The Problem

In a 2004 editorial in the Journal of American College of Cardiology, Sylvan Lee Weinberg, former president of the American College of Cardiology and outspoken proponent of the diet-heart hypothesis, said:

"The low-fat, high-carbohydrate diet... may well have played an unintended role in the current epidemics of obesity, lipid abnormalities, type 2 diabetes, and metabolic syndromes. This diet can no longer be defended".

Simply put, if you add cholesterol to a cholesterol-free diet, the blood levels will go up *for a short period of time*, but they *go back down to normal* as soon as your body gets used to the change in diet.

WHAT ABOUT BUTTER

Despite being blamed for everything from obesity to heart disease in the past few decades, butter has been making a comeback as a healthy choice recently. Here's why:

Butter is Good For You. This does not mean you can slop it on with a trowel, but it is *a better choice than margarine.*

Butter is Rich in Fat-Soluble Vitamins

Butter contains several fat soluble vitamins including vitamins A, E and K2.

Vitamin K2 is fairly rare in the modern diet and it can have powerful effects on your health. It's involved in calcium metabolism and a low intake has been associated with many serious diseases, including cardiovascular disease, cancer and osteoporosis.

Dairy from grass-fed cows is particularly rich in Vitamin K2.

Butter Contains a Lot of Healthy Saturated Fats

The war against saturated fat was based on bad science, meaning it was never really proven that it was harmful. Recent studies suggest there is no association at all between saturated fat and cardiovascular disease.[4]

Saturated fats raise HDL (the good) cholesterol and change the LDL from small, dense (very bad) to Large LDL, which is benign.

Additionally, butter contains short and medium chain fats which are metabolized differently from other fats that lead to improved satiety and increased fat burning.

Butter Lowers Heart Attack Risk Compared to Margarine[5]

Due to nutrition guidelines, many people replaced butter, a healthy food, with something containing highly processed trans fats. This type of advice is as bad as it gets.

The current understanding is that margarine raises the risk of heart attack while natural butter does not. In fact, butter from grass-fed cows may even reduce heart attack risk due to the high Vitamin K2 content.

Butter is a Good Source of The Fatty Acid Butyrate

The 4-carbon fatty acid butyrate is created by bacteria in the colon when they are exposed to dietary fiber, and this is one of the main reasons fiber has health benefits for humans.

Butter contains about 3-4 percent butyrate and butyrate derives its name from butter.

In humans, butyrate is anti-inflammatory and produces protective effects on the digestive system.[6]

Butter is Rich in Conjugated Linoleic Acid

Butter, especially grass-fed, is a great source of a fatty acid called Conjugated Linoleic Acid. This fatty acid is actually sold commercially as a weight loss supplement.

CLA has been shown to have anti-cancer properties as well as lowering body fat percentage in humans.[7]

NOTES

[1] US National Library of Medicine – "Meta-analysis of prospective cohort studies evaluating the association of saturated fat with cardiovascular disease" (http://www.ncbi.nlm.nih.gov/pmc/articles/PMC2824152/)

[2] Harvard School of Public Health – "Fats and Cholesterol: Out with the bad: In with the good" – (http://www.hsph.harvard.edu/nutritionsource/fats-full-story/)

[3] (http://www.nutritionjrnl.com/article/S0899-9007%2811%2900314-5/fulltext)

[4] US National Library of Medicine – "Meta-analysis of prospective cohort studies evaluating the association of saturated fat with cardiovascular disease" (http://www.ncbi.nlm.nih.gov/pmc/articles/PMC2824152/)

[5] http://www.fasebj.org/content/early/2000/12/02/fj.00-0359fje.long

[6] (http://ar.iiarjournals.org/content/26/1A/27.long)

[7] IJCRT "Conjugated Linoleic Acid (CLA) Up-regulates the Estrogen-regulated Cancer Suppressor Gene, Protein Tyrosine Phosphatase Á (PTPÁ), in Human Breast Cells" (http://ar.iiarjournals.org/content/26/1A/27.long)

CHAPTER 7

Glycemic Index and Glycemic Load

Carbohydrates used to be classified as simple or complex based on the number of simple sugars in the molecule.

We were told to eat fewer simple carbs based on the assumption that starchy foods caused smaller increases in blood glucose than sugary foods. It turns out it's not that simple.

If the food has a low glycemic index and a low glycemic load, it is more likely to be burned as fuel. If the food has a high glycemic index and a high glycemic load, it is more likely that it will be stored as fat.

The glycemic response relates to how any food affects these three areas:

1. Does it raise blood glucose levels
2. Does it increase the release of insulin
3. Does it stimulate Lipoprotein Lipase (LPL) and fat storage

---

HOW IT'S CALCULATED

Using pure glucose as a standard with an index of 100, scientists compare how a 50 gram portion of various carbohydrates affect blood sugar compared to pure glucose and rate the carbohydrates on a scale from 0 to 150.

Foods that are lowest on the glycemic index have the slowest rate of glucose entry into the bloodstream, and therefore have the lowest insulin response.

Glycemic Index Guidelines	
Low (good)	0 - 55
Medium (acceptable)	56 - 70
High (avoid)	70 +

The Glycemic Index (GI) tells you how rapidly certain foods affect your blood glucose within 2-3 hours. Here's a chart that shows the glycemic index of a few vegetables you might have as a snack:

Glycemic Index for Vegetables - 100g	
Vegetables	Glycemic Index
Bell Pepper	10
Broccoli	10
Carrot	35
Cauliflower	15
Celery	15

The glycemic index tells us that carrots have a greater effect on your blood sugar levels than celery or broccoli. It gives us more information than the traditional simple vs complex carbs approach, but it still does not give us enough information.

The Glycemic Load goes one step further and gives you the impact of a given serving and also takes fiber into account. Here's how it's calculated:

Glycemic Load Calculation			
Glycemic Load =	Glycemic Index / 100	x	Net Carbs
* Where net carbs = Total Carbs - Fiber			

Glycemic Load Guidelines

And here's the glycemic load for the same vegetables that we saw in the glycemic index chart:

Glycemic Load for Vegetables		
Vegetables	Serving Size	Glycemic Load
Bell Pepper	92g (1 cup sliced)	2
Broccoli	91g (1 cup chopped)	3
Carrot	122g (1 cup strips)	3
Cauliflower	100g (1 cup)	2
Celery	64g (1 stalk)	1

As you can see, we get a different picture once we take fiber into account. The glycemic load chart provides much more useful information than the glycemic index chart did.

Carrots appeared to be a worse choice than the other vegetables according to the glycemic index, but when we look at the glycemic load, we see that all of these vegetables are in the low range and they are all very good choices.

It's important to realize that the serving size affects the glycemic load rating. Generally speaking, if you double the serving size, the glycemic load will double as well.

However,

The Glycemic Load doesn't tell you that a food is good to eat!

The glycemic load provides useful information but it is not a good indicator of *which* foods you should eat. For example, Frosted Flakes may have a lower GL than many fruits, but natural fruit is obviously a better choice.

Which Index Should I Use

It's important to realize that neither index tells you anything about the quality of food.

Both the glycemic index and the glycemic load provide valuable information. However, they both have shortcomings. The glycemic index might sway you to avoid foods that are good to eat while the glycemic load could make you think it's ok to eat foods you should avoid.

Here's how I use them:

I try to avoid high glycemic index foods or at least limit how much of them I eat. The glycemic load of those foods helps me understand the impact of serving size.

For example, carrots have an average glycemic index of 35 (20 raw and 50 boiled) and a glycemic load of 3. Sweet potatoes have a glycemic index of 70 and a glycemic load of 22.

With this information, I know I don't have to worry about carrots, even when boiled. Also, most of us are not inclined to have a huge serving of carrots.

Sweet potatoes on the other hand, are something we need to be concerned about. Both the glycemic index and the glycemic load are high. What's worse is that many of us can eat a large sweet potato in one meal!

When I have a sweet potato, I have a very small one, or half of a medium sized one, and I don't have them more than once or twice a week.

By considering both the glycemic index and the glycemic load in this way you can make informed choices about your food selections. If you are only going to pay attention to one of them, focus on the glycemic load.

Sugar Substitutes

There is no question that refined sugar and high fructose corn syrup (HFCS) are incredibly bad for your health. The question is, what is safe to use to sweeten your food and beverages?

Artificial Sweeteners

In one study, 3,682 people were examined over 7-8 years for the long-term relationship between consuming artificially sweetened drinks and weight.

After adjusting for common factors that contribute to weight gain such as dieting, exercise or diabetes status, the study showed that *people who drank artificially sweetened drinks had a 47 percent higher increase in BMI* (weight) than those who did not use artificial sweeteners.[1]

Natural Sweeteners

Natural sweeteners like agave may seem like a healthier choice, but they're loaded with fructose and many are also highly processed. Because *fructose is the worst offender when it comes to sugars,* agave is probably a poorer choice than pure table sugar.

Agave syrup has more fructose content than any commercial sweetener at over 70 percent. HFCS, in comparison, average 55 percent fructose. Agave nectar or syrup is laboratory-generated super condensed fructose syrup.

Honey also averages about 53 percent fructose, but unlike agave, it is completely natural in its raw form, and has many health benefits when used in moderation. Remember that most commercial Grade A honey is highly processed and of poor quality and what you want is raw, natural honey.

Problems With Refined Fructose

Refined fructose (as opposed to natural) turns off your body's appetite-control system. Fructose does not appropriately stimulate insulin, which in turn does not suppress ghrelin, the hunger hormone, and doesn't stimulate leptin, the satiety hormone, which together result in your eating more and developing insulin resistance.[2]

Fructose activates a key enzyme that causes cells to store fat; this is the fat switch discussed in Dr. Richard Johnson's book.

Refined fructose leads to weight gain and abdominal obesity, decreased HDL, increased LDL, elevated triglycerides, elevated blood sugar, and high blood pressure, all of which characterize the classic metabolic syndrome.

Finally, refined fructose eventually contributes to insulin resistance, which is an underlying factor of type 2 diabetes and heart disease.

Sugar Alcohols

Sugar alcohols like xylitol, glucitol, sorbitol, maltitol, mannitol, glycerol and lactitol can be identified by the 'ol' at the end of their name. They're not as sweet as sugar and they do contain fewer calories. Labelling rules allow for some foods sweetened with sugar alcohols to have the sugar-free label.

Sugar alcohols are not completely absorbed by your body. While this provides fewer calories, it can lead to abdominal gas and diarrhea.

Safe Sugar Alternatives

Stevia

This is the sweetener that I use. Stevia is derived from the leaf of the South American stevia plant and is sold as a supplement. It is completely safe in its natural form and can be used to sweeten most dishes and drinks.

You want to buy a powdered form that is made from the entire stevia leaf because it's the synergistic effect of all the agents in the plant that provide the overall health effect, which often includes built-in protection against potentially damaging effects from ingesting concentrated isolated ingredients of the plant. Unfortunately, what the FDA has approved as GRAS (generally recognized as safe) are just a couple of the active ingredients, like rebaudioside A, and this is what the large commercial producers are using.

Rebaudioside A

In a toxicology review of rebaudioside A by Sarah Kobylewski and Curtis D. Eckhert, Ph.D., the researchers pointed out that stevioside compounds and rebaudioside A are metabolized at different rates.

In other words, studies show that taken as a whole, stevia is non-toxic, but we cannot say the same about isolated rebaudioside A with certainty just yet. They concluded that separate toxicity studies on rebaudioside A are necessary to make definitive conclusions about its safety for long term use.

Type of Stevia To Buy

Try to find stevia rebaudiana powder made from the entire leaf and not just a concentrate of one of the active ingredients. There are roughly 200 varieties of stevia, but *stevia rebaudiana is the sweetest variety and it does not have the bitterness that many complain of* when using stevia.

Lo Han Kuo

Lo Han Kuo is another natural sweetener similar to Stevia, but it's a bit more expensive and harder to find. In China, the Lo Han fruit has been used as a sweetener for centuries, and it's about 200 times sweeter than sugar. It received FDA GRAS status in 2009.

Glucose

If you don't want to give up sugar and you don't have much of a weight problem or insulin resistance, a third alternative is to use pure glucose. It is more expensive than sugar and is not as sweet as sucrose, but it is a healthier alternative as it does not contain any processed fructose.

Glucose can be used by every cell in your body, however, it is best to stick to stevia if you have a weight problem.

WHY USE STEVIA

Stevia is very sweet and it has virtually no calories.

There are some studies in humans showing Stevia to have health benefits. When blood pressure is high, Stevia can lower it by 6-14 percent. However, it has no effect on blood pressure that is normal or only mildly elevated. Stevia has also been shown to lower blood sugar levels in diabetics

Stevia has also been shown to improve insulin sensitivity, reduce oxidized LDL cholesterol and reduce plaque build-up in the arteries in rats.

Stevia is probably the healthiest choice in sweeteners available to us today. While some people hate the taste of stevia, I'm sure it's because they used the wrong kind. Buy an extract of pure stevia rebaudiana; it is very sweet and does not taste bitter if you use a bit too much.

How To Buy Stevia

Stevia is a natural, zero-calorie sweetener that can lower both blood pressure and blood sugar levels. The key is to buy pure stevia. As with most things, you need to beware of gimmicky labeling tactics. There are many stevia products are available but many come with fillers and additives.

The best choice is *a powdered product that is 100 percent pure stevia extract*. Beware of stevia powder which indicates a blend and not pure extract. Pure stevia isn't cheap but it goes a long way since a tiny pinch is as sweet as a teaspoon of sugar.

You can find pure stevia in health food stores and sometimes in a grocery store's organic section. Be sure to read the ingredient list and if you see anything except 'pure stevia extract', keep looking!

Notes

[1] Harvard School of Public Health "Artificial Sweeteners" (http://www.hsph.harvard.edu/nutritionsource/healthy-drinks/artificial-sweeteners/#ref56)

[2] JAMA and Archives Journals. "Fructose has different effect than glucose on brain regions that regulate appetite." (www.sciencedaily.com/releases/2013/01/130101182010.htm)

CHAPTER 8

EXERCISE

Is it necessary to exercise to lose weight? Will you be able to keep the weight off if you don't exercise?

Many clinical trials have been carried out by researchers to find out which combination of weight loss program works best in the treatment of obesity:

- Diet only
- Exercise only
- A combination of diet and exercise.

As expected, the groups that used a combined program of diet and exercise always lost the most weight.

However, exercising alone without proper nutrition often does not work, especially for obese individuals.[1]

WHY EXERCISING ALONE DOESN'T WORK

People often eat the wrong types of food after exercising and they end up just replenishing the calories and glycogen that was burned during the exercise session.

During exercise, people use the glycogen stored in the muscle and liver as their main source of fuel. If you eat a meal that is high in carbs, the glycogen that was burned during exercise will reform. Even if you work out again the next day, only the newly formed glycogen will be used instead of the stored fat.

The result is that stored fat is rarely burned up in exercise only programs. Exercise without the right diet will not burn fat unless you exercise many hours a day, every day. For this reason, exercise alone is not really the answer to weight loss for most people[2].

THE DIET ONLY OPTION

A diet only option will allow you to lose a significant amount of weight providing you eat the right foods.

You won't lose weight as fast as you would if you were exercising as well, but you can still lose a significant amount of weight without breaking a sweat.

Having said that, exercise will help you lose weight more quickly and you should get involved in physical activity to whatever extent you can. If you can only manage to go for a brisk walk, do it!

Not only will it help you lose weight more quickly, it will boost the function of your lymphatic system.

Benefits of Exercise

Regular exercise speeds up your metabolism, which means you will use more energy in any given time than you would were you not exercising. You will also increase your lean muscle mass which also helps burn more fat.

In addition, exercising improves the movement of your lymphatic system and makes you feel better by enhancing the production of natural opioids.

The increased circulation boosts oxygen to the brain which will improve your mental ability. Generally speaking, your general health and well-being will improve with your level of activity.

Unless you have a health condition which makes it hard for you to exercise, it's really just a matter of changing your habits a bit to create a new routine.

NOTES

[1] PMC "Why do individuals not lose more weight from an exercise intervention at a defined dose? An energy balance analysis" D.M. Thomas et. Al.
(http://www.ncbi.nlm.nih.gov/pmc/articles/PMC3771367/)

[2] Plos "Changes in Weight, Waist Circumference and Compensatory Responses with Different Doses of Exercise" Timothy S. Church
(http://journals.plos.org/plosone/article?id=10.1371/journal.pone.0004515)

CHAPTER 9

WHY DIETS FAIL & HOW TO SUCCEED

The average person gains about 10 pounds for every diet they go on. What's worse, when they lose weight, they lose muscle and fat and when they put the weight back on, *it's all fat.*

The typical diet only makes their problems worse because their metabolism ends up slower than it was when they started the diet, and the muscle they lost burned several times more calories than the fat gained!

> *They need even fewer calories to maintain their weight than they did before the diet.*

WHY MOST DIETS FAIL AND HOW TO SUCCEED

Some Diets Use a Non-Scientific Approach

The diets that suggest you eat less actually trigger hunger.

You can only starve yourself for so long before your famine survival mechanism compensates to protect you from starvation, even if it is self-induced as in a strict low-calorie diet.

Your hunger increases dramatically, your cravings go up and your metabolism slows down, all to conserve energy. By eating certain foods with low fat and higher carbs or sugary foods, you actually increase hunger and slow your metabolism.

How To Succeed: *Don't Eat Less – Eat Different*

- Eat enough whole fresh food to satisfy your appetite.
- Eat protein for breakfast and try to avoid eating 3 hours before bedtime.
- Eat meals designed to balance blood sugar and prevent insulin spikes.
- Combine protein and low-glycemic carbs at each meal. Fat, protein and fiber slow insulin spikes.

- Don't mix carbs and high fat foods especially during a weight loss phase.

Focusing on calories (the eat less do more plan)

The mantra of calories in/calories out or energy balancing as the key to weight loss does not take advantage of the knowledge that is available to us today.

All calories are not created equal in the sense that some make you fat and some make you thin. Any foods that spike insulin will trigger a shift in your metabolism making insulin drive most of the fuel in your blood from the food you just ate into your fat cells.

How To Succeed: *Eat low glycemic carbs with protein or fiber*

- Make very low-glycemic foods the staples of your diet. Nuts, chicken, fish, grass fed meats, organic dairy and eggs, low-glycemic veggies, salads etc.
- Eat grains sparingly.
- Avoid sugar of any kind. I only use pure Stevia to sweeten things (and a bit of pure maple syrup on occasion).
- Don't use artificial sweeteners.

Eating a High Carb Low Fat Diet

The fact that fat has 9 calories per gram and carbs and proteins have 4 calories per gram led to the disastrous idea that we could lose weight by eating more carbs and less fat.

The results of this experiment are easily visible. The rate of obesity keeps rising and nearly 70 percent of the population is considered to be overweight.

Walter Willet from Harvard reviewed the science and found that it is not fat that makes you fat but carbohydrates.

A study by David S. Ludwig, MD, PhD and others shows that *by eating more fat and fewer carbs you can increase your metabolism by 300 calories a day.*

That's the equivalent of running for an hour a day without getting off the couch! (http://jama.jamanetwork.com/article.aspx?articleid=1199154)

How To Succeed*: *You Need Good Fats

- Fat makes you feel full and it speeds up your metabolism which helps you lose weight.
- Eat good fats often.
- Eat vegetable fats like nuts, seeds, coconut butter or olive oil.
- Eat clean animal fats like organic eggs with the yolk, organic chicken, grass-fed meats and fish like sardines, herring, wild salmon and cod.

Eating Foods That Cause Inflammation

Inflammation can be caused by food intolerance or food allergies (people often become intolerant to foods they eat too often).

Gut Problems. The bacteria in your gut play an enormous role in metabolism and health. Eating the wrong foods can either trigger inflammation or alter how your food is broken down and absorbed.

Toxins. Common environmental chemicals like pesticides, household cleaners, make up, pollution and heavy metals can be 'obesogens' (chemicals that make you fat). Scientists found that giving rats a toxin caused weight gain even if they ate the same amount of calories and exercised the same.

How To Succeed: *Find Hidden Causes of Weight Gain*

- *Try an elimination diet*: Eliminate inflammatory foods from your diet for a few weeks and see if you feel different.
- *Fix your gut:* Avoid acid blockers, antibiotics and anti-inflammatories. Starve the bad bugs by eating a low-glycemic, low-fermentation diet. Take probiotics.
- *Detox your body:* Reduce your exposure to environmental and common chemicals. Stop eating highly processed food.

The Famine Survival Mechanism

One of the main reasons most diets fail is because of the body's 'famine survival mechanism'. It's a survival system that activates a series of physiological mechanisms that help protect us from losing too much weight too quickly.

In pre-agricultural times, which take in the majority of human history, the food supply was sporadic and depended on weather, the seasons and your ability to hunt. Conserving energy ensured survival through the lean season.

But while our famine survival mechanism helped the species survive recurring famines and hardships, it presents an enormous challenge in modern societies where there is abundance of food and the option to make many bad food choices.

The famine survival mechanism is a whole-body response to not getting enough food.

It creates three main symptoms:

Hunger – when you start a weight-loss program, you might not feel very hungry at all. But once you lose a certain amount of weight, you might suddenly find that you are still hungry after eating your regular meals. That's the famine survival mechanism pushing you to eat more to help protect you from losing any more fat.

Lethargy – once you've lost weight and your famine survival mechanism gets activated, you will feel sluggish. It's as if you have to drag your body around through the day. You're being slowed down so you don't waste precious energy and lose any more fat.

Reduced Metabolic Rate – you feel cold and shivery, even in the middle of summer. This is your famine survival mechanism reducing your metabolic rate. It's one of the reasons you come to a plateau or standstill in your weight loss, even though you are sticking to your diet and exercise plan.

Fighting the famine survival mechanism

Research shows that the changes that accompany the famine reaction don't just stop when you stick with your diet.

The only way to neutralize this mechanism is to eat more so your body thinks the famine is over.

You have to work with your physiology, not against it. This means eating when you're hungry.

By eating a bit more and entering a period of weight maintenance, you can deactivate some aspects of the famine survival mechanism.

This process can take place quite naturally when you hit plateaus in your weight loss journey. Don't panic or get discouraged when this happens. *Most importantly, don't cut your food intake!* Just be careful of what it is you eat. The plateau will come to an end and you will resume losing weight.

Once you understand this, you won't get disappointed at each plateau you reach. In fact, you should think of it as a necessary step to go through before you shed a few more pounds!

CHAPTER 10

Inflammation & Weight Control

Weight loss is NOT just about calories. It's about controlling hormones like insulin, cortisol, leptin and decreasing inflammation.

There's a connection between food allergies, inflammation and weight problems. If you eat foods that you are intolerant or allergic to, it causes inflammation which makes your adrenal glands secrete hormones that destabilize your insulin and blood sugar levels.

A high level of insulin affects the activity of enzymes which cause your body to hold on to and deposit fat rather than allowing you to burn it for energy. So food allergies can lead to weight gain, and a high amount of body fat can promote inflammation and worsen problems with allergies.

Fat Cells and Inflammation

Any excess body fat also contributes to inflammation. When you gain weight, your body doesn't create more fat cells. Your existing fat cells stretch as they are filled with more fat and they can leak as they get stretched more and more. When this happens, immune cells called macrophages begin cleaning up the mess by releasing inflammatory chemicals in the fatty tissues.

In response, cells release anti-inflammatory chemicals that can interfere with the function of the hormone leptin. In healthy people, leptin is responsible for automatically maintaining weight at the right level.

Some people don't gain weight no matter what they eat. When they overeat, their leptin control system boosts their metabolism and decreases their appetite to restore them to their best weight.

As leptin is made ineffective by inflammation, a dysfunction called leptin resistance develops, and your leptin stops working to suppress your appetite and speed metabolism.

The good news is that as you slim down, your leptin resistance decreases and your system goes back to work controlling your appetite and weight as it should.

Reducing Inflammation

You can reduce inflammation by watching the type of fat you consume.

Prostaglandins are made from the fats we eat. Some prostaglandins promote inflammation and some reduce it. The essential omega-3 fatty acids eicosapentaenoic acid (EPA) and docosahexaenoic acid (DHA) help the production of anti-inflammatory prostaglandins.[1]

Most people don't eat enough fish to produce the omega-3 fatty acids they need and can benefit from fish oil supplementation.

Some foods like ginger, cherries, blueberries, other dark berries, pomegranates, and some fruits and vegetables also have anti-inflammatory properties. Add some of these foods to your diet to help control inflammation.

Probably the best way to reduce inflammation is to stabilize and reduce insulin levels.[2]

Inflammation can have many causes including allergic reactions, asthma, arthritis, inflammatory bowel disease etc. You can minimize inflammation by following a healthy eating plan that controls your blood sugar, taking fish oil supplements and eating anti-inflammatory foods.

Two Simple Changes

There are two simple changes to your diet that will improve your health and control inflammation:

1. Eat in a way that eliminates blood sugar and insulin spikes and maintains insulin at a relatively constant low level.
2. Include a generous amount of anti-inflammatory foods in what you eat.

Notes

[1] Your Hormones "Prostaglandins" (http://www.yourhormones.info/hormones/prostaglandins.aspx)

[2] Foodallergy.org "Allergies, Inflammation and Weight Control" (http://www.food-allergy.org/inflammation.html)

CHAPTER 11

YOUR LYMPHATIC SYSTEM

Your lymphatic system supports every other system in your body, including the digestive, immune, detox and nervous systems. *Poor lymph health underlies a number of conditions from cellulite to cancer.*

You have twice as much lymph fluid as you do blood. Lymph fluid continuously bathes each cell in your body and drains away the debris. There's no pump in your lymph system; it's powered by your breathing and movement.

> *You would die within hours if the movement of the lymph stopped completely.*[1]

ANATOMY OF THE LYMPH SYSTEM

The network of lymph vessels serves your entire body. Lymph nodes are strung along lymph vessels and work as a series of cleaning filters.

As the lymphatic fluid percolates through the nodes, it is purified and immunologically boosted. Lymph tissue also stores the white blood cells that fight infection.

Digestive Function

The largest concentration of lymph tissue in the body surrounds the intestines and is called gut-associated lymphatic tissue, or GALT.[2]

Your GALT guards the largest gateway through the body's defenses by separating desirable nutrients from undesirable pathogens (infectious agents) and it helps mount a defense whenever needed.

THE FLOW OF LYMPH FLUID

Your cells use nutrients and excrete waste. There may be pathogens or antigens present that create an immune response leaving dead cells and sometimes live infection. This process is happening all over your body all the time.

One blocked lymph node can be bypassed, but when blockage is extreme it causes the lymph fluid to back up and create swelling in the surrounding tissue, a condition known as lymphedema.

Your lymph fluid also backs up when it gets blocked due to toxic overload and/or lack of activity.

This can cause swelling, joint pain, nausea and fatigue

Eventually, stagnant lymph becomes too toxic for the body to handle and can cause a number of problems.

Chronic Lymph Blockages

Your lymph system could be compared to a river. A healthy river runs clean and clear, while a brackish river chugs along, thick with filth and silt that gets snagged and creates pockets of pollution along the way. Eventually, the sluggish river becomes a breeding ground for bacteria and disease. The same is true for your lymph.

Symptoms of chronic lymph blockage are many and include:

- Allergies and food sensitivities
- Frequent cold and flu infections
- Swelling and joint pain
- Headaches and migraines
- Arthritis
- Fibrocystic breasts and breast tenderness
- Fatigue, mental fuzziness and depression
- Parasites, skin breakouts, acne, and cellulite.

THE LYMPHATIC SYSTEM, DIGESTION AND ELIMINATION

Your eating habits can expose you to offensive substances like bacteria, allergens, heavy metals, molds, fungi, chemicals and trans fats.

Your GALT receives information from the intestines as to which pathogenic agents get through. It then decides which of these deserve an allergic response and calls on the immune and endocrine systems to respond. This is one of the reasons why the gut is called the second brain.

The healthier your gut-associated lymph tissue is, the less sensitive you are to food-borne bacteria and chemicals.

The lymphatic system and cellulite

Cellulite and saddle bags along the thighs are partially caused by the impaired lymph flow to those areas which causes pockets of fat and trapping of toxins.

Fat cells collect in one area and cause the skin to bulge. Toxins and lymph fluid then accumulate in the pockets of fat.

You can reduce cellulite by improving the circulation of lymph in those areas and by reducing the toxic burden on your system.

Lymphatic massage

Inactivity can seriously restrict the flow of lymph. Exercise and deep breathing are the primary means by which our lymph circulates, but lymphatic massage and drainage provide another helpful option.

How To Improve Your Lymphatic System

- ***Reduce the toxic burden:*** Avoid processed food and eat organic whenever possible. Reduce or eliminate simple sugars and high glycemic carbs.
- ***Take supplements:*** Take a good multivitamin and probiotic supplements to help maintain a healthy ratio of intestinal flora.
- ***Drink lots of purified or filtered water:*** Drink six to eight 8oz glasses per day.
- ***Practice deep breathing:*** Breathing deeply from the diaphragm is one of the best ways to move lymph fluid through your body.
- ***Exercise regularly:*** Find an activity that suits you. What's important is that you make it a regular and fun part of your life.
- ***Sweat:*** Take a weekly sauna or steam bath. Avoid aluminum-based antiperspirants and use a natural deodorant instead.
- ***Be Happy:*** Stress and boredom slow down your lymph system. Move and enjoy life.

NOTES

[1] Merk Manuals – "Overview of the Lymphatic System" (http://www.merckmanuals.com/professional/cardiovascular_disorders/lymphatic_disorders/overview_of_the_lymphatic_system.html)

[2] Anatomy Atlases – "Lymphatic System" (http://www.anatomyatlases.org/MicroscopicAnatomy/Section09/Section09.shtml)

CHAPTER 12

Processed Foods

The word *processed* often causes some confusion, so let's define it as it relates to our food.

Most of the foods we eat are processed in some way. Apples are picked from trees, ground beef has been ground in a machine and butter is cream that has been separated from the milk and churned. These are examples of mechanical processing.

What Are Processed Foods

There is a difference between *mechanical* processing and *chemical* processing.

If the food has no added chemicals, it doesn't matter if it's been ground or put in a jar. It's still real food.

However, when foods have been chemically processed and made mostly from refined ingredients and artificial substances, they are generally known as *processed food*.

Processed Foods Are Usually High in Sugar and High Fructose Corn Syrup

---

Why You Should Quit Eating Processed Foods

Sugar and HFCS

Most processed foods are loaded with added sugar or High Fructose Corn Syrup (HFCS). Many studies show that sugar has devastating effects on our metabolism that go way beyond its calorie content. Sugar consumption can lead to insulin resistance, high triglycerides, increased levels of harmful cholesterol and increased fat accumulation.

If you're trying to lose weight, sugar is one of the first things you should limit in your diet.

And where does most sugar consumption come from? It's from processed foods and sugar-sweetened beverages.

Overconsumption

It's human nature to want to eat. We naturally crave foods that are sweet, salty and fatty because we know these foods contain energy and nutrients that we need for surviv-al.

Manufacturers compete for our food dollars and massive resources are spent on making foods as desirable as possible.

As a result, many processed foods have been engineered to be so incredibly rewarding to your brain that they create stronger cravings than anything you would come across in nature.

This high reward value leads us to eat more than we need, to the point that our health can be compromised. This is also known as the 'food reward hypothesis of obesity.'

Foods that are engineered to short-circuit your innate mechanism against overconsumption are NOT good.

Artificial Ingredients

If you look at the ingredients label on many processed foods, chances are you won't know what many of them are. That's because many of the ingredients aren't actual food but artificial chemicals that are added for various purposes.

Even products that are marketed as 'healthy diet products' are manufactured in this manner. For example, here's the ingredients list for a 'diet' food called the Atkins Advantage bar:

Nutrition Facts
Serv. Size 1 Bar (60g)

Amount Per Serving	
Calories 250 Fat Cal. 120	
	% Daily Value*
Total Fat 14g	22%
Saturated Fat 8g	40%
Trans Fat 0g	
Cholesterol <5mg	1%
Sodium 190mg	8%
Potassium 110mg	3%

INGREDIENTS: CHOCOLATE FLAVORED COATING [POLYDEXTROSE, PALM KERNEL AND PALM OIL, WHEY PROTEIN ISOLATE, COCOA POWDER (PROCESSED WITH ALKALI), SOY LECITHIN, ARTIFICIAL FLAVOR, SUCRALOSE, ACESULFAME POTASSIUM], PEANUT BUTTER FLAVORED LAYER [MALTITOL, PALM KERNEL AND PALM OIL, PEANUT BUTTER, PARTIALLY DEFATTED PEANUT FLOUR, NONFAT DRY MILK, WHEY POWDER, PEANUTS, SALT, SOY LECITHIN, ANHYDROUS MILK FAT, COCOA POWDER (PROCESSED WITH ALKALI)], GLYCERIN, PROTEIN BLEND (SOY PROTEIN ISOLATE, WHEY PROTEIN ISOLATE, SODIUM CASEINATE), PEANUTS, HYDROLYZED GELATIN, WATER, POLYDEXTROSE, PEANUT BUTTER (GROUND, ROASTED PEANUTS), CELLULOSE, NATURAL AND ARTIFICIAL FLAVORS, PALM KERNEL OIL, OLIVE OIL, CLARIFIED BUTTER, SOY LECITHIN, GUAR GUM, VITAMIN MINERAL MIX [DICALCIUM PHOSPHATE, MAGNESIUM OXIDE, ASCORBIC ACID (VITAMIN C), SODIUM ASCORBATE, VITAMIN E ACETATE, NIACINAMIDE, ZINC OXIDE, D-CALCIUM PANTOTHENATE, PYRIDOXINE HYDROCHLORIDE (VITAMIN B6), THIAMIN MONONITRATE (VITAMIN B1), RIBOFLAVIN (VITAMIN B2), VITAMIN A PALMITATE, FOLIC ACID, BIOTIN, CHROMIUM AMINO ACID CHELATE, SODIUM SELENITE, PHYLLOQUINONE (VITAMIN K1), CYANOCOBALAMIN (VITAMIN B12)], SALT, MALTODEXTRIN, CITRIC ACID, SUCRALOSE, MONO AND DIGLYCERIDES, DIPOTASSIUM PHOSPHATE. FR02
CONTAINS PEANUTS, SOY AND MILK.
THIS PRODUCT IS MANUFACTURED IN A FACILITY THAT USES OTHER NUTS, SEEDS AND WHEAT.

Even if you do manage to lose weight eating products like this, imagine the long term health effects from eating this stuff every day. This is not real food!

MSG

Monosodium Glutamate (MSG) is approximately 78 percent glutamic acid and 22 percent sodium. It is an excitotoxin that makes you think the food has more protein and tastes better by tricking the tongue using a fifth basic sense called umami.

Some of the adverse effects linked to MSG are obesity, headaches, fatigue and disorientation and depression.

MSG Symptom Complex

MSG symptom complex includes symptoms such as numbness, facial pressure or tightness, chest pain or difficulty breathing, headache, nausea and rapid heartbeat.

While food manufacturers have to list MSG as an ingredient, they do not have to label ingredients that contain free glutamic acid, which is the main component of MSG!

List of ingredients that *ALWAYS* contain MSG:

Ingredients That Always Contain MSG		
Autolyzed Yeast	Calcium Caseinate	Gelatin
Glutamate	Glutamic Acid	Hydrolyzed Protein
Monopotassium Glutamate	Monosodium Glutamate	Sodium Caseinate
Textured Protein	Yeast Extract	Yeast Food
Yeast Nutrient		

Here's a list of ingredients that *OFTEN* contain MSG:

Ingredients That Often Contain MSG		
Flavor and Flavoring	Soy Protein Isolate	Pectin
Stock & Broth	Maltodextrin	Barley Extract
Malt Extract/Flavor	Citric Acid	Enzymes
Protease	Soy Protein Isolate	Bouillon
Seasonings Soy Sauce	Pectin Powdered Milk	Corn Starch Carrageenan
Natural Chicken Flavoring	Anything Enzume Modified	Anyting Protein Fortified

The best way to avoid MSG is to pay attention when reading labels and limit how often you eat out. Good home cooked meals are the only way to know what it is you are eating!

Lack Of Nutrients

Processed foods are low in essential nutrients despite the fact that some manufacturers add synthetic vitamins and minerals to make up for what was lost during processing.

Synthetic nutrients are NOT equivalent to the nutrients found in whole foods because they lack the trace elements and complimentary nutrients that are necessary for the body to absorb and utilize the vitamins and minerals.

Lack Of Fiber

Natural fiber is often lost or intentionally removed during processing. This eliminates the benefits of fermentable fiber which acts as a prebiotic that stimulates the growth of good bacteria in the bowel.

Fiber slows down the absorption of carbohydrates, helps us feel more satisfied and also helps prevent constipation.

Bad Fats

Processed foods are usually high in unhealthy fats. They're usually made with refined seed and vegetable oils that are hydrogenated, a process which turns them into trans fats.

The seed oils are extracted from crops like Soybean, Cottonseed and Sunflower etc. and are manufactured using a harsh extraction process that includes bleaching, deodorizing and a highly toxic solvent called hexane.

Unsuspecting consumers are being duped into buying all sorts of *supposedly healthy foods* like salad dressings, butter substitutes, mayonnaise and diet cookies that contain these products.

GMOs

GMO's were first introduced into our food supply in the mid-1990's and are now present in the vast majority of processed foods in North America. The two main traits that have been added to date are herbicide tolerance and *the ability of the plant to produce its own pesticide.*

Where Are GMOs

Currently commercialized GMO crops include over 90 percent of crops like soy, cotton, canola, sugar beets, corn and some of the Hawaiian papaya, zucchini and yellow squash.

From these crops, manufacturers derive other products like oils, soy protein, soy lecithin, cornstarch, corn syrup and high fructose corn syrup among others.

Should You Avoid GMOs

You can find strong opinions on both sides of this argument and it would take another book to do the subject justice.

But considering that GMO foods typically contain considerably more pesticide residue, I prefer to purchase organic hands down. Granted organic foods do cost more to purchase, and if you're on a limited budget, you should choose based on the issue of pesticide residue.

Do they make a difference as far as weight loss goes? Not likely, especially in the short term.

I personally find a huge difference between GMO or mass-produced foods vs organic or small scale home-grown style foods when it comes to taste. Frankly, the mass-produced/GMO foods have little to no flavor in comparison to organic or fresh out of your garden crops!

CHAPTER 13

Reading Food Labels

Many of the better choices for a healthy diet have no labels at all. Most whole foods, what some call *real food* don't come with a label.

These include vegetables, meats, fruits, and other fresh foods that have all of their nutrients intact, and are usually low in sugars and starches. There are some whole foods with labels, like nuts and frozen vegetables.

As a general rule, it's best to stay away from packaged foods as much as possible.

That said, there is a lot of information on nutrition labels to help us understand what's in the food we eat. Some parts of the label are confusing and need special attention. So let's start to understand how to read nutrition labels, with a focus on the carbohydrate content of labels.

Serving Size

You need to pay special attention to the serving size section of the label. It's important to understand that a serving size may have little to do with the amount of the food most of us eat as a 'serving'.

Next, there's the issue of rounding error. When a label says that 1 tablespoon has one gram of carbs, there could be anything from .51 grams to 1.49 grams because that represents the allowable error due to *rounding.*

That's not a big deal if you're only eating one serving. But if the serving is one tablespoon, and you're going to use a cup in your recipe, you need to adjust for the fact that there are 16 tablespoons in one cup. The rounding error could be as much as 8 grams in either direction.

> ***That means there could be anywhere from 8 grams to 24 grams of carbs in that one cup serving!***

CHAPTER 14

ELH DIET - PHASE 1 RESET

How To Get Off The Merry-Go-Round

To break the cycle created by craving bad foods, you need a change in lifestyle.

By doing this, not only will you change *what* you eat but *what you crave to eat*. And that's the biggest hurdle for many people. When the cravings for bad foods are gone, it won't be so hard to keep your weight in check.

Luckily, there is a way to do this in as little as one week!

THE 3RS OF THE ELH DIET

Phase 1 – Reset

We reset our systems in one week of strict food intake. This breaks the food addictions and poor eating routines we've become stuck in.

Phase 2 – Retrain

We retrain ourselves with new eating habits during the second phase. As we add foods back into our diet, we pay attention to any food sensitivities we may have. This is the secondary and main weight-loss phase.

Phase 3 – Retain

We continue our new dietary lifestyle and retain our new base line weight. We carry on with the easy, lean and healthy dietary lifestyle, but now that we've reached our target weight, we don't have to be as strict with our food choices. If we happen to wander off the path the odd time, we might gain a lb. or two, but this won't be a big deal because we will be used to having our weight vary within a 1 to 3 lb. range already.

WHAT'S DIFFERENT ABOUT THIS APPROACH?

Rather than trying to lose weight by eating less, you will just eat differently. It's more of a change in lifestyle than a diet. And, once you've made the adjustment, you won't feel deprived because *you will no longer crave* the unhealthy foods that caused your weight problem.

The main difference with this approach is that you will be working with your biological system, rather than against it.

- You can eat anytime you get hungry.
- Exercise is good, but you don't have to.
- You don't have to count or worry about calories.
- Fats are not taboo.
- You will break your addiction to sugar and junk foods.
- You will gradually repair insulin & leptin resistance.
- You stop fighting a losing battle with processed foods.

Your taste buds will come back to life and you'll start enjoying food again!

It's Not All About The Calories

While it is true that consuming more calories than you expend will lead to weight gain, it does not follow that all calories are the same.

ALL CALORIES ARE NOT CREATED EQUAL

A recent study challenged the notion that 'a calorie is a calorie' when it comes to the human diet. The study "Effects of Dietary Composition on Energy Expenditure During Weight-Loss Maintenance" by Cara B. Ebbeling, PhD et. Al. concluded that all calories are not created equal.[1]

David Ludwig said "We've found that, contrary to nutritional dogma, all calories are not created equal".

Dr. Cara Ebbeling led the trial of 21 overweight and obese participants aged 18-40, and found that resting energy expenditure and total energy expenditure were reduced more with a low-carbohydrate and/or a low-glycemic index diet, *even though all participants consumed the same amount of calories.*

Dr. Ebbeling said that "Total calories burned plummeted by 300 calories on the low fat diet, which would equal the number of calories typically burned in an hour of moderate-intensity physical activity".

In other words:

If you increase the amount of good fats you eat (or get off the low fat bandwagon) you will automatically start burning extra calories, equivalent to about 1 hour of moderate exercise every day!

The Study Compared Three Diets:

1. A low-fat diet of 60 percent calories from carbohydrates, 20 percent from fat and 20 percent from protein. This is the Standard American Diet (SAD).

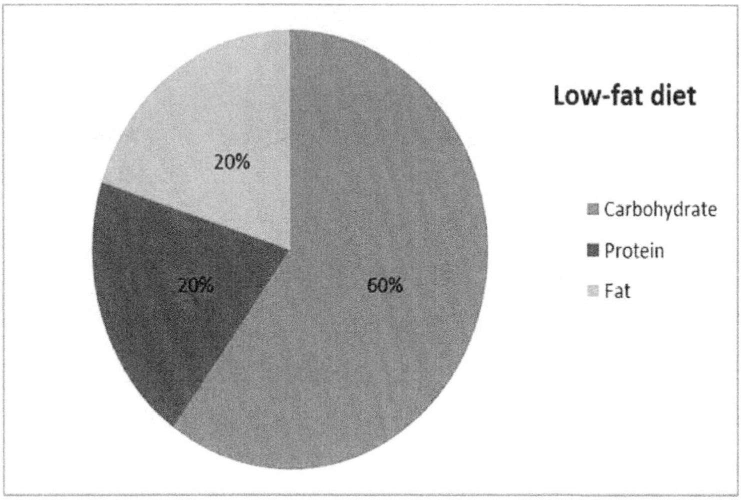

Many people think this low fat/high carb diet has inadvertently contributed to the obesity epidemic. As fats were removed from processed and prepared foods, most food producers substituted added sugar to improve the bland taste that resulted from removing natural fats.

2. A very low-carb Atkins style diet of 10 percent calories from carbohydrates, 60 percent from fat and 30 percent from protein.

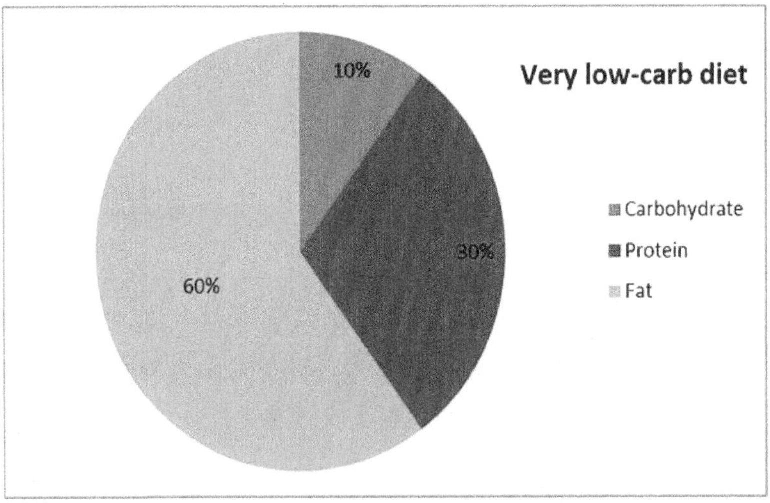

3. A low-glycemic index diet of 40 percent calories from carbohydrates, 40 percent from fat and 20 percent from protein.

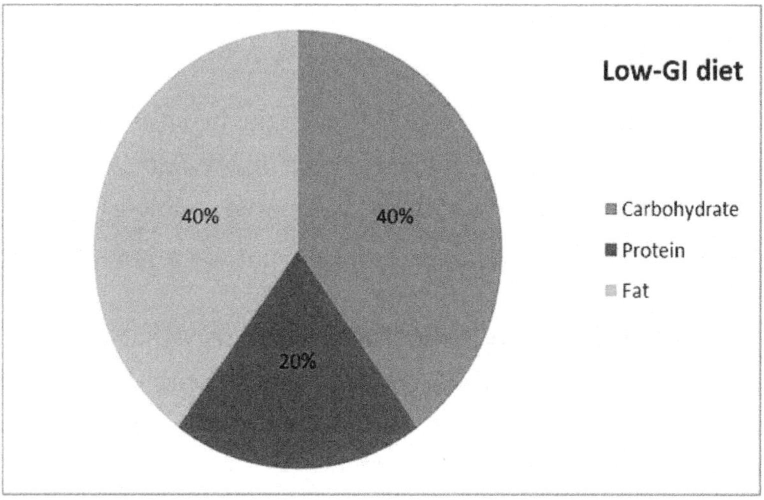

Results showed that each diet does affect metabolism and components of the metabolic syndrome in noticeably different ways, independent of the energy content.

The recommended low-fat or SAD diet (Standard American Diet), produced changes in energy expenditure and serum leptin that would predict weight regain. In addition, this conventionally recommended diet had unfavorable effects on most of the metabolic syndrome components.

While the very low-carbohydrate (Atkins style) diet produced the best results on energy expenditure and several metabolic syndrome components, it had minor side-effects in that it increased cortisol excretion and CRP slightly.

The winner was a low–glycemic index diet. It was almost as effective as the very-low carb diet and is more balanced and easier to follow.

Dr. Ebbeling added "In addition to the benefits noted in this study, we believe that *low-glycemic index diets are easier to stick to on a day-to-day basis*, compared to low-carb and low-fat diets".

These findings suggest that a diet strategy that reduces glycemic load along with a moderate increase in dietary fat is beneficial for weight-loss, weight maintenance and cardiovascular disease prevention.

We're aiming for the sweet spot between diet #2 and diet #3.

By simply removing sugar and reducing your intake of processed foods from your diet, you will reduce your carbohydrate intake significantly.

You then take it one step further by eating a low glycemic load diet. When you do eat carbohydrates, you eat them with roughage or protein to achieve a lower glycemic load. Finally, by increasing your intake of good quality fats, you hit the sweet spot in diets.

It's Not A Good Idea To Eat Less

There's no doubt that a low calorie diet can help you lose weight in the short term. The problem is, as you cut down your calorie intake by eating less, *your body adjusts and will need less food to function going forward.*

The longer you cut down your food intake, the less food your body needs. So, *a reduction in calorie intake today becomes tomorrow's normal intake.*

The minute you come off that diet, not only will you spring back up to where you were, but you will put on even more weight because your body needs fewer calories to function now than it did before you went on the diet!

You now have to eat less just so you don't put on weight!

That's a guaranteed recipe for failure over the long term and it's probably why people who go on diets end up gaining weight over the years!

USE A LOW GLYCEMIC LOAD APPROACH

We pay close attention to the glycemic load of foods. Why? Because it's our insulin and leptin levels that affect weight gain more than anything else.

Glycemic Load Guideline

Glycemic Load Guidelines	
Low (good)	0-10
Medium (acceptable)	11-19
High (avoid)	over 20

Here's how it works:

When you eat carbs, they get converted to sugars, your blood sugar level goes up and your body produces insulin to return your blood glucose level back to the safe range it was in before you ate the carbohydrates.

Foods that cause a large and rapid glycemic response cause a boost in energy and mood as your blood sugar rises. Unfortunately, they also increase fat storage and a cycle of lethargy, and more hunger!

The glycemic load tells you how much effect any particular food will have on your blood sugar level. For instance, meat has a glycemic load of zero because it doesn't cause your body to produce any extra insulin, unless you are diabetic.

If you focus on eating foods with a glycemic load of less than 15 and eat your carbohydrates with roughage or protein, you will avoid producing insulin spikes and storing extra fat.

Is That All You Have To Do?

Unfortunately, no. Most of us have developed poor eating habits and have developed strong cravings for foods that encourage weight gain. We need to reset our systems. The first week of the ELH diet will help you do this and put an end to craving foods you should be avoiding. We do need to be aware of the glycemic load of the foods we eat, but that's just part of what we need to do.

The ELH Diet

In order to get off this crazy treadmill, we need to understand what it is that's been causing our problems.

It really boils down to just a few things:

- Stop poisoning yourself – quit eating sugar.
- Use stevia to sweeten foods and drinks.
- Quit eating processed foods and junk food.
- Avoid mid to high-glycemic load carbohydrates.
- Limit your intake of carbs to match the phase you are in.
- Eat low-fat protein with your fruit.

During phase 1, eat only the foods that are listed in the chart below. If it's not there, don't eat it.

That's pretty much it! Sounds simple doesn't it?

Reset

Why We Need Phase 1 – Reset

Many things in modern day life need to be reset occasionally. With computers, we reset them by rebooting the system. We do that by stopping whatever programs are running and reset the system by stopping it and then starting it back up again.

Similarly, we need to *reset* our systems occasionally. This is what Phase 1 is all about.

We need to go through phase 1 for a couple of reasons. First, we need to change our eating habits. And because our commitment is always highest in the first couple of weeks when trying something new, we're going to take advantage of this and use it to cut out unhealthy foods and see whether or not we have become intolerant to some of the foods we eat.

Second, we want to lose weight, and you should lose 4-5 lbs. during this phase. This weight loss will boost your incentive to stick with the diet and help you lose even more weight during the second phase.

We're going to get off to a running start in our weight loss program by taking a very strict approach at the beginning.

For the first five to seven days, you will give up sugar, fruit, grains, high glycemic foods and most processed foods as well. We only eat certain things to kick start our weight loss program.

Most of you will lose 4-5 lbs. in the very first week of this diet. You will also take a big step in breaking free from the hold food cravings have on you.

PHASE 1 – WEEK 1

Phase 1 - Week 1	
Things You Can Eat	**Things You Can't Eat**
Fish	Deserts (cake, biscuits, jams)
Meat	White rice, processed foods
Eggs, olive oil, butter	Fruit juices, soft drinks, milk
Yogurt	Fruits, grains
Vegetables, cooked mushrooms	Cheese, pickled foods
Brown rice in moderation	Potatoes
Water *(tea, coffee, alcohol)	Note*

*Ideally, we would add alcohol, tea and coffee to the list of *things you can't eat* in the first week.

If you can manage to cut these out, all the better. I've left them in because I don't want the diet to be so restrictive it discourages anyone from trying the diet.

However, this first week does present a great opportunity for anyone who would like to deal with all of these habits at once.

Alcohol in particular should be used in moderation during this first week.

INSTRUCTIONS

In the first five to seven days, eat only the foods that are listed in the chart. There is no restriction on how much you eat.

You can eat as much as you want of anything on the list *except* for the brown rice, which needs to be limited to a small serving. Don't let yourself get hungry because that will only lead you to reach for something to snack on that might not be on the list.

Another reason to not let yourself get hungry is that it will kick in your body's *famine survival mechanism.*

Some people need to start the day with a good breakfast that sticks with them like ham and eggs or an omelet. That's a great breakfast and you can keep doing that. The only thing you must leave out is the toast (carbs) and jam (sugar) that you might normally have for breakfast. You can add field tomatoes for a bit more variety.

You'll be amazed at the taste of food after the first few days. Once you cut out sugar and highly processed foods you will start to taste the natural sugar and sweetness that is in so many things.

You will be surprised at how sweet many foods are once you're no longer de-sensitized to natural sugars

I should mention that you might feel some detox-like symptoms from cutting out carbs and as your body rids itself of all the junk that's in the processed foods you've been eating. Most people usually feel better at the same time, but you could feel a bit disoriented or foggy headed.

That's why it's a good idea to start phase 1 on a Wednesday or Thursday, so you get through most of it by the following Monday.

Listen To Your Body

Pay attention to any strong food cravings you get during this first week. These cravings will most likely come from foods you eat often and have developed an '*intolerance*' to.

By the end of the week, these cravings will have subsided considerably if not entirely.

Food Intolerance

When you develop intolerance to a certain food, your digestive system does not produce enough enzymes to completely break it down into smaller components.

The unabsorbed food becomes a meal for the bacteria in your digestive tract and you suffer symptoms like gas, bloating, tummy cramps and in some cases diarrhea. Pay attention when this happens and avoid any foods that cause this type of response.

Make a note of which foods don't agree with you. Any slight intolerance to a food can lead to inflammation and contribute to weight gain by causing fluid retention and a host of other issues.

* One important point to note is the Ebbeling/Ludwig study did not have any participants that fit the definition of very obese or suffering from metabolic. For these individuals, it has been shown that the very low-carb diet is the preferred route to weight loss, at least in the early stages.

This isn't going to be the most exciting week you've had in terms of food choices, but it will do what it is intended to do. Stick with the program, you won't be sorry!

NOTES

[1] · JAMA "Effects of Dietary Composition on Energy Expenditure During Weight-Loss Maintenance" Cara B. Ebbeling, PhD et. Al. (http://jama.jamanetwork.com/article.aspx?articleid=1199154#RESULTS)

CHAPTER 15

ELH DIET - PHASE 2 RETRAIN

Congratulations! You've made it through the first week of the program and hopefully, you've lost more weight than you thought you could possibly lose in one week!

You're probably also looking forward to having a bit more variety in your diet!

> *According to Webster, to retrain means 'to train again or anew' and appetite is defined as 'a physical desire for food'. These two definitions fit perfectly with what we intend to accomplish in this portion of the diet.*

It is our appetite for certain foods that needs to change in order for us to reach our goal. We often become so set in our eating habits that we can't imagine changing our diet (what we eat). It's really not that difficult. You're half way there right now!

EXPANDING YOUR FOOD CHOICES

In this second phase of the diet you get to eat a larger variety of food, but you still need to be careful about blood glucose levels and always try to minimize the glycemic load of anything you eat.

We continue to avoid sugar and highly processed foods. This is simply the easiest way to cut down on calories *without cutting down on food.* You should stay on this phase until you reach your target weight.

You need to eat when you are hungry. Don't make the mistake of starving yourself with small portions in an effort to lose weight more quickly. This approach is guaranteed to backfire because your body will learn to get by on fewer calories.

PLATEAUS

If your goal is to lose a lot of weight, you will no doubt hit several plateaus on your journey. Remember this is normal, just keep going and you *will* get there.

Not only will you hit plateaus, your weight might even vary within a range of 1-3 pounds within any given week. Mine does exactly that!

WHAT DO I EAT?

Personally, I don't eat a large breakfast in the morning. I usually have fruit and yogurt when I get up and I often have a second serving a couple of hours later.

Or, I might have some cottage cheese with fruit rather than yogurt. We're all different and you need to tailor the diet in a way that works for you.

I have a larger meal for lunch, usually eggs in an omelet or hard-boiled, what others may have had for breakfast. Another choice I often have for lunch is something left over from last night's dinner, especially if it was a stir fry.

You can have whatever you like whenever you like, provided the food is on the 'foods you can eat list'.

My largest meal is in the evening and it's not much different than what I used to eat, minus the potatoes or rice. I have some meat (chicken, beef or pork) and at least 2 large servings of vegetables. Rather than potatoes or rice, I sometimes have a third type of vegetable.

I do have potatoes and rice once or twice a week, but it's always a small serving, just to add variety to the diet.

Things to remember about this part of the program:

Any food that you really crave at this point is something you've probably developed intolerance to. Try not to eat anything you *really* crave too often until you break the craving.

- Don't eat sugar.
- Don't eat junk food or fast foods.
- Don't eat processed foods.
- Avoid high glycemic load carbohydrates.
- Eat your carbs with roughage or protein if possible.

Keep eating your fruit with low-fat protein whenever you can, and don't mix higher glycemic carbohydrates and high-fat proteins during the weight loss period. The higher the glycemic index of any carbohydrate, the more you need to keep this in mind. Carbs drive insulin levels up and any dietary fat is more likely to be stored in your fat cells.

Processed Foods

You need to stay on a diet of good, natural foods as much as possible. Remember that most snack foods are processed; chips, crackers and dried fruit are all processed foods.

However, if you're like most people, you usually can't get everything fresh or organic. Just remember that when you do buy something that is in a package or a can, read the ingredients and avoid anything with sugar and/or chemical additives. Try to buy the most natural products you can find.

Carbohydrates and Fatty Foods

Because this is a weight loss phase, we try to eat our carbohydrates with very low fat protein. Eating some protein with your carbs helps you reduce the amount of carbs you eat and also helps you feel full for a longer period of time.

Remember, carbs and sugars drive insulin levels up and makes your body store fat.

Don't cut your food intake or your body will go into famine survival mode and will store fat *even if you cut your calorie intake.*

HOW MANY CARBOHYDRATES

The latest US dietary guidelines issued in 2010 recommend that adults get 45-65 percent of their daily caloric intake from carbohydrates!

This might be an ok recommendation for extremely active individuals, but for anyone who is overweight and trying to lose weight, this is way too much.

Unless you decide to have some surgically removed, the only way to lose body fat is to burn it. If you go back to Chapter 4 and review the information on ketosis, you will see that you need to reduce your carbohydrate intake to below 100 grams per day if you want to seriously burn fat.

You need to reduce your daily intake of carbohydrates if you want to burn body fat

Categorizing Foods

CATEGORIZE FOODS
Anything you eat falls into one of these categories
Carbohydrates
Protein
Fats

You need to categorize any food you eat to help you plan your meals and snacks. Why?

Because *your body is always looking to burn whatever is easiest to convert to energy, and that's carbohydrates.* So if you eat any carbs that are not very low glycemic index with fats or high-fat protein, your body will burn the carb portion and store some of the fat! You're can't lose weight when you do this; you might gain some though.

Keep in mind that we're not talking about tiny amounts of carbs or fats. For example, even though there's a bit of fat in low fat cottage cheese, it's ok to eat it with carbohydrates. In fact, it's a good way to reduce the glycemic load of whatever carb it is you are eating. But don't have a toasted cheese sandwich because bread is high glycemic and there is too much fat in regular cheese.

Three Food Categories:

High Fat Protein Meals	Carb Meals
Meat: Beef, pork, chicken etc..	Grains: Cereal, bread, fruit, pasta, rice
Dairy: Cheese	Baked potatoes (unpeeled)
Low Fat Protein Meal	
Fish: Fresh or tinned (in water or oil)	Beans: Chickpeas, lentils etc..
Dairy: Low fat milk, cheese, yogurt	
Fats	
Butter, oils	

What About Protein?

All protein contains a certain amount of fat. We need to think of some protein sources as being in the high-fat category, so we eat them with few or no carbohydrates, especially during a weight loss phase.

You can eat low fat protein, like fish, skim or low fat cottage cheese anytime you like. It's good to do this as you will feel more satisfied for a longer period and you will also eat fewer carbohydrates in that meal or snack.

Chicken breast baked with skin on is about 8 percent fat, and that's why it's considered a high-fat protein while we are in a weight-loss phase.

Whatever category foods fit into, make sure you buy unprocessed foods. For meats, that means fresh cuts of beef or pork. There should be no other ingredients on the package.

For breads and cereals, make sure there's no sugar of any kind and choose whole grain. Shredded Wheat is one of the few big name brand cereals that does not have sugar or additives.

For rice or pasta, choose whole grain brown rice and whole wheat pasta.

*** Allow 3 to 4 hours after a carb-rich meal before you eat a high-fat meal and vice versa.

Neutral Foods

Luckily many foods are very low glycemic and/or very low fat and that means we can eat them anytime with any other food.

Here's another chart for you to print off and keep handy:

Neutral Foods That Go With Any Category	
Vegetables	
Salad Ingredients	Celery, cucumbers, green onions, kale, lettuce, radishes, tomatoes, spinach, swiss chart etc..
Raw or cooked with meals	Asparagus, beets, broccoli, brussel sprouts, cabbage, chic peas, eggplant, garlic, onions, peppers, turnip etc..
For stir fries	Bamboo shoots, celery, bean sprouts, bok choy etc..
Low Fat Dairy	
Cottage cheese, milk, yogurt	

These neutral foods go with any meal and give us a break from the strict regime that makes up most diets. For example, you can use hummus, a chick pea spread, on toast to replace jam or peanut butter.

It's important to eat three regular meals a day and not let yourself get hungry from not eating enough. You will lose weight no matter how much you eat on this diet provided you always minimize the glycemic load of things you eat.

HOW MUCH WEIGHT CAN YOU EXPECT TO LOSE?

Most people can expect to lose 4-5 lbs. in the first week, but some might lose more than that. By the end of the first month, you can expect to lose between 10 to 20 lbs. on this diet. These are pretty good results when you consider that you can eat as much as you want.

Each of us has a different activity level, our own rate of metabolism and we each make different food choices. That's why we all get different results. Chances are that you'll lose as much or more weight than you did on any other diet you've tried in the past.

The Long Haul

More importantly, you'll be dealing with what's been causing you to crave 'junk foods' and getting rid of the insulin spikes that cause weight gain in most people. If you stick to your new dietary lifestyle, you will NOT regain the weight later on.

SALT

Remember to keep an eye on your salt consumption. If you happen to eat a lot of salt, your body will retain more water and you probably won't lose weight as fast as you would if you had reduced your salt consumption a bit too.

Salt is also on the list of ingredients that boost the 'pleasure response' of foods. That means it can lead to overeating.

WHAT ABOUT SNACKS?

This is a tough one for many people and it's probably one of the areas that contribute the most to weight gain. Some of the usual culprits are chips, dry roasted peanuts and sweets of any kind.

All of these snacks need to be eliminated because they are processed foods and most contain sugar.

Hummus

Veggies and hummus are my go-to snack. Hummus provides a combination of plant protein, unsaturated fat, fiber, iron, zinc, magnesium and folate.

It can serve as a dip or spread that is vegan-friendly, gluten-free and suitable for guests with common food allergies. Hummus can be used as a binder for tuna, chicken or egg salad, a coating for baked chicken breasts; a topping for baked potatoes.

Peanuts in the Shell

Peanuts in the shell are also a good snack; they're a natural food packed with nutrition. Some people do have allergies or sensitivities, so be aware. As with any other food, it's best if you can find organic peanuts.

Keep in mind that a snack is supposed to be just that – a snack. A heaping plate or a huge bowlful of something is not a snack. Remember always that *actions you repeat will eventually become habits.*

Here's what's in one cup of shelled peanuts:

Nutrional Summary for One Cup of Shelled Peanuts			
Calories	Fat	Carbs	Protein
305	26.8g	7.8g	14g
Calorie Breakdown	73%	9%	18%

Remember this is for one cup of *shelled peanuts*. You will be consuming considerably far fewer calories in one cup of raw peanuts in the shell.

Peanuts are high in calories and contain fat, carbs and protein. If you were on a calorie counting diet, you would probably not eat them, and would instead choose a processed, low-fat diet snack in a misguided effort to lose weight.

But peanuts are a natural food that is packed full of great nutrients including, oleic acid, quality amino acids, resveratrol, vitamin E, and many important B-complex groups of vitamins such as riboflavin, niacin, thiamin, pantothenic acid, vitamin B-6, and folates.

Peanuts are a rich source of minerals like copper, manganese, potassium, calcium, iron, magnesium, zinc, and selenium. That's spells a good, healthy snack, and unless you happen to be allergic to them, they're probably one of the best snack foods you will find.

Peanuts are also satisfying because of the high fat content. Remember, fat makes you feel full.

Fruit as a Snack

Fruit such as apples, pears, berries and peaches make a great snack. If you eat them with a bit of protein they can be quite filling as well.

During this period of weight loss, limit yourself to two to four pieces of fruit per day. Not only are fruits carbs, they also contain natural sugars. I usually cut my fruit into a serving of low fat yogurt to make the snack more nutritious and more filling.

FOR THE SWEET TOOTH

I hate to break the news, but deserts and weight loss don't play well together. My go-to treat is a small handful of grapes. They will give you a natural sugar fix and deliver some good nutrition at the same time. Don't over indulge!

You can also have the occasional piece of dark chocolate. Buy 90 percent pure chocolate to reduce the amount of sugar – the chocolate itself is good for you. It will probably taste a bit bitter at first, but it will taste pretty sweet once you get used to it.

Remember to mix very low fat proteins like yogurt or cottage cheese with carbohydrates. This lowers the glycemic load, makes your snacks more filling *and* will satisfy your hunger for a longer period of time.

When cooking, use Stevia to sweeten. When you have the urge to be a bit more decadent, you can use a *small amount* of pure maple syrup (real maple syrup from a market).

WHAT ABOUT EATING OUT?

To many people, eating out means eating at one of the many fast food restaurants. As a rule, these foods are not that different from the highly processed foods you buy at the grocery store as far as the impact on your diet and health.

If you happen to eat out while you're in this weight-loss phase, the best choice to make is to choose foods that fall in the protein category and some neutral class foods. They may not be as unprocessed as you would like, but it will be a better choice than whatever carbohydrates might be on the menu.

Pay attention to how you feel afterwards. Once you've been off the processed food diet for a while, you will notice that you don't feel so well after eating these foods. You might even feel a bit ill or bloated afterwards.

HORMONES RULE

You will notice that as you lose weight, your body resists and keeps trying to put the fat back on. If you check your weight regularly, you will probably see your weight move up and down in a 1 to 3 lb. range within any given week!

Don't get discouraged, this is quite normal as you establish a new baseline level of body fat

LEPTIN AND INSULIN – THE HORMONAL DANCE

Leptin and insulin work together to regulate energy intake and energy expenditure. A resistance to either hormone is associated with obesity.

Insulin and leptin both have an effect on the quality of your metabolism and your rate of metabolism.

What Exactly is Leptin?

Leptin is a hormone that is produced by your fat cells. Your fat, by way of leptin, tells your brain whether you should be hungry and eat to make more fat. Leptin is the way that your fat stores speak to your brain to let your brain know how much long-term energy is available and what to do with it.

In a normal individual, when your fat storage is full, there is a surge in leptin that signals your brain to stop feeling hungry so you stop eating. It also tells your brain to stop storing fat and to burn extra fat off.

Controlling your hunger signal is the main way that leptin controls energy storage. It's what keeps you from eating too much to the point that you get fat!

How You Become Leptin Resistant

Like insulin resistance, leptin resistance develops as your system continuously pumps out too much leptin.

When you eat a diet that is high in sugar, grains, and processed foods, these foods are broken down into sugar which gets metabolized in your fat cells. As the fat builds, more and more leptin gets released.

As your body gets exposed to too much leptin over time, it becomes resistant or numb to the signal and quits sending out the *you're full, you can stop eating now* message it would normally send out.

The only way we know of to re-establish proper leptin and insulin signaling is to prevent the surges in hormone by controlling what you eat. What you eat has repercussions far beyond your weight.

CHAPTER 16

ELH DIET - PHASE 3 RETAIN

You should have reached your target weight by now. Congratulations! Now you can relax your diet a little and you don't need to worry so much about mixing carbohydrates and high-fat protein in the same meal.

Webster defines the word retain as 'to continue to have'. This suits the last phase of our program because it is exactly what we intend to do in regards to our weight.

Whether it took three months or six months, you're back to a happy weight and you can finally fit into the clothes you've only been able to watch hang in your closet for a long time.

Things You Need To Keep Doing

- Don't eat sugar
- Don't eat processed foods
- Be careful if you add back any food that you had a food addiction to before going on the diet.
- Keep avoiding high GI foods as much as possible.

The easiest way to keep the weight off going forward is to relax your diet just a little bit. Don't go crazy and think you don't have to be concerned about what you eat now that you've reduced your weight!

Remember, people often fool themselves into thinking they can eat anything after coming off a diet. They gorge themselves and because extra weight doesn't come on right away, they start thinking that their metabolism has changed and they've suddenly become immune to weight gain. Duh!

The truth is, the weight might not show for a few days or weeks, but *you will put it back on if you persist in eating the wrong foods!*

Keep Up The Good Habits

You want to keep whatever good eating habits you've been using. For example, keep eating your fruit with a low fat protein to help make you feel full and keep your insulin from spiking.

When you have an apple, orange or fruit of any kind, try cutting it up and putting it in a serving of natural (sugar-free) yogurt. Eating protein with carbs will help keep your blood sugar from spiking and keep you feeling full for a longer period of time.

Don't go back to eating junk food. It's all highly processed food and it will lead you right back into being a food addict again. It taxes your lymph system, causes inflammation and makes you feel ill.

If You Fall Off The Wagon

There will no doubt be times when you have to eat out, or perhaps not be able to follow the diet as closely as you'd like for a few days. When you do eat a high glycemic load food, remember to eat some fiber or protein with it to keep your blood sugar from spiking so much – and try to keep the portions small.

This isn't a trick that will allow you to gorge yourself on high GL foods, but it will help a bit on those occasions.

GROCERY SHOPPING

Fats

Now that you've reached your target weight, you shouldn't have to worry about buying low fat milk cottage cheese, regular cheese or yogurt.

Try to buy organic or at least dairy from grass fed cows if you can. Animals that eat a natural diet have a healthier fat that is rich in omega 3 fats rather than omega 6.

GLYCEMIC INDEX & LOAD CHARTS

Here are a few charts showing the nutritional composition, glycemic load and the glycemic index of some common foods. This information will help you make food choices based on the proportion of carbohydrates, fat and protein as well as the glycemic load.

Remember that the glycemic load is just part of the information you should use in choosing foods. It does not tell you whether any particular food is a good choice. Let's look at a typical hot dog for example:

Junk Food	CARBS	FAT	PROTEIN	GL	SERVING
Frankfurter (beef & pork)	2%	82%	16%	0	45g (1)
A & W Hot dog	29%	55%	16%	11	90g (1)

The frankfurter by itself has few carbs and a zero glycemic load, as do most meats.

Even after adding the bun as in this plain hot dog from A & W (I don't mean to single them out, I'm sure you'll get basically the same nutrients wherever you go) we see it falls within acceptable limits as far as carbohydrate or glycemic load.

But we all know it's not good food!

However, the information is useful to help us compare foods that we know are good for us. Remember to stick to your new eating habits. It's the easy way to be lean and healthy!

Glycemic Load And Glycemic Index Charts

FOODS

VEGETABLES (boiled)	CARBS	FAT	PROTEIN	GL	SERVING	GI
Beans gr	80%	7%	13%	4	115 g (1cup)	30
Beans yel	80%	7%	13%	4	125g (1 cup)	30
Broccoli	73%	10%	17%	4	140g (1 sm stalk)	15
Brussel sprouts	71%	12%	17%	3	100g (2/3 cup)	15
Cabbage gr	82%	6%	12%	1	35g (1/2 cup)	15
Cabbage red	85%	4%	11%	1	35g (1/2 cup)	15
Celery (raw)	73%	10%	17%	0	64g (1 lg stalk)	15
Celery (cooked)	82%	7%	11%	2	75g (1/2 cup)	35
Carrots (raw)	90%	4%	6%	2	78 g (1/2 cup)	20
Carrots (cooked)	90%	4%	6%		78 g (1/2 cup)	40
Corn on the cob	82%	10%	8%	**20**	150g (2 reg ears)	**65**
Peas gr	76%	2%	22%	4	78 g (1/2 cup)	**55**
Potatoes white	92%	1%	7%	**21**	140g (~ 1 sm)	**70**
Potato sweet (baked)	94%	1%	5%	**22**	140g (~ 1 sm)	**70**
Potato russet (baked)	88%	1%	11%	**33**	140g (1 sm)	**111**
Tomato	79%	9%	12%	2	1 lg (3" dia)	45
Zucchini	87%	3%	10%	1	90g (1/2 cup)	15

FRUIT	CARBS	FAT	PROTEIN	GL	SERVING	GI
Apple	95%	3%	2%	6	149g (1 sm)	35
Banana (raw)	93%	3%	4%	**16**	100g (1 sm)	**55**
Grapefruit	90%	3%	7%	3	118g (1/2 cup)	25
Grapes	94%	2%	4%	11	151g (1 cup)	45
Olives gr	10%	88%	2%	0	6g (3 olives)	0
Olives ripe	20%	78%	2%	0	8g (2 lg olives)	
Oranges (navel)	91%	3%	6%	5	140g (1 med)	45
Pears	96%	2%	2%	5	148g (1 sm)	15
Peach	87%	5%	8%	5	130g (1 sm)	**50**

BEANS, NUTS & OTHER	CARBS	FAT	PROTEIN	GL	SERVING	GI
Beans baked	56%	30%	14%	6	150g (2/3 cup)	30
Beans kidney	49%	15%	36%	7	150g (1/2 cup)	30
Cashews	23%	68%	9%	**15**	137g (1/2 cup)	25
Chick peas	68%	13%	19%	3	150g (2/3 cup)	35
Chick peas (canned in brine)	78%	8%	14%	9	150g (2/3 cup)	35
Hummus	35%	48%	17%	0	61g (1/4 cup)	25
Peanuts (valencia)	15%	70%	15%	0	50g (1/3 cup)	25
Peanut butter - no sugar	15%	71%	14%	0	32g (2 Tbs)	**50**
Pistachios	20%	67	13	5	123g (1cup)	15
Mushrooms (br. Roasted)	50%	18	32	1	56g (1/2 cup)	**70**

BEVERAGES	CARBS	FAT	PROTEIN	GL	SERVING	GI
Apple juice (unsweetened)	97%	2	1	**30**	250ml (1 cup)	44
Orange juice (unsweetened)	91%	4%	5%	12	250ml (1 cup)	**50**
Tomato juice	87%	2%	11%	4	250ml (1 cup)	38

GRAINS & CEREALS	CARBS	FAT	PROTEIN	GL	SERVING	GI
Whole wheat bread	66%	14%	20%	10	2 slices	**71**
Whole wheat bread	66%	14%	20%	**20**	4 slices	**71**
Bread rye	77%	11%	12%	**16**	2 slices	
Bread bran	75%	12%	13%	**18**		
Rice brown	85%	7%	8%	16	150g (3/4 cup)	**50**
Rice white (avg)	90%	2%	8%	**43**	150g (3/4 cup)	**89**
Rice Uncle Ben's Converted	88%	3%	9%	14	150g (3/4 cup)	38
Shredded Wheat Post	85%	3%	12%	24	50g (1 cup)	**75**
Shredded wheat & bran	81%	4%	15%	26	60g (1 cup)	**75**
Oatmeal	79%	7%	14%	30	250g (1 cup)	**83**
Oatmeal (instant - cooked)	71%	17%	12%	30	250g (1 cup)	**83**

PASTA & NOODLES (boiled)	CARBS	FAT	PROTEIN	GL	SERVING	GI
Spaghetti white	81%	5%	14%	22	180g (1 1/4 cup)	46
Spaghetti whole wheat	81%	4%	15%	**15**	180g (1 1/4 cup)	46

MEAT - R (roasted) P (pan fried)	CARBS	FAT	PROTEIN	GL	SERVING	GI
Beef roast (R)	0%	34%	66%	0	200g	0
Beef reg ground (P)	0%	60%	40%	0	113g (1/4 lb)	0
Beef lean ground (P)	0%	54%	46%	0	113g (1/4 lb)	0
Chicken with skin on						
Chicken roasted (R)	0%	51%	49%	0	100g (2/3 cup)	0
Chicken breast (R)	0%	36%	64%	0	100g (2/3 cup)	0
Chicken breast (F)	3%	36%	61%	0	100g (2/3 cup)	0
Chicken drumstick (R)	0%	47%	53%	0	100g (2/3 cup)	0
Chicken drumstick (F)	2%	51%	47%	0	100g (2/3 cup)	0
Chicken with skin off						
Chicken roasted (R)	0%	35%	65%	0	100g (2/3 cup)	0
Chicken breast (R)	1%	23%	76%	0	100g (2/3 cup)	0
Chicken drumstick (R)	0%	30%	70%	0	100g (2/3 cup)	0
Pork roast	0%	56%	44%	0	450g (1lb)	0
Port cutlet (center cut)	0%	37%	63%	0	170g (6 oz)	0
Port back ribs	0%	72%	28%	0	220g (1 lb)	0

EGGS & DAIRY	CARBS	FAT	PROTEIN	GL	SERVING	GI
Egg (hard boiled)	3%	62%	35%	0	2 lg	0
Egg (fried)	2%	70%	28%	0	1 lg	0
Egg (scrambled)	5%	66%	29%	0	2 lg	0
Egg (omelet)	2%	69%	29%	0	2 lg	0
Egg (poached)	2%	63%	35%	0	2 lg	0
Cheese cottage	13%	39%	48%	4	113g (1/2 cup)	0
Cheese cottage 2%	16%	25%	59%	4	113g (1/2 cup)	0
Cheese cottage 1%	15%	12%	73%	6	113g (1/2 cup)	0
Milk 3%	30%	49%	21%	5	1 cup	41
Milk 2%	39%	25%	26%	5	1 cup	39
Milk 1%	46%	20%	34%	5	1 cup	36
Milk skim	56%	5%	39%	4	1 cup	32
Yogurt reg plain	29%	47%	24%	4	113g (1/2 cup)	35
Yogurt low fat plain	42%	22%	36%	10	113g (1/2 cup)	35
Yogurt reduce fat w fruit avg	73%	10%	17%	11	245g (1 cup)	33

Sticking With Your New Diet

There's a reason why diets fail and people regain lost weight plus a few extra pounds.

Some diets set you up for failure simply because they cause changes to your metabolism which cause you to gain weight as soon as you come off the diet. You will come off the diet if it's not something you can stick with long-term.

Weight loss that lasts is based on changes you can live with for a long time.

The ELH Diet allows you to eat lots of really good food. All you've had to give up is junk food, fast foods and prepared foods. If you think about that for a minute, you'll realize the only thing you've given up is stuff you shouldn't have been eating in the first place.

Parting Words

The ELH Diet allows you to eat lots of really good food. The junk foods and processed foods you've given up are not natural, healthy food. These foods are manufactured for one reason; to get you to eat more than you should as a way to increase corporate profits.

The secret to long-term weight loss is changing your appetite – what it is you crave to eat. If you've made it this far, you have changed your appetite and your eating habits. All you need to do going forward is stick to your new routine.

Habits aren't made overnight, so if you happen to stray off the path for one meal, make sure it's only once so you don't fall back into a bad eating pattern.

When you eat out, eat protein and low glycemic carbs and don't eat sugar filled food of any kind. You've kicked that addiction, why would you go back. You wouldn't have a cigarette after quitting smoking would you?

If you have questions or need a bit of encouragement in your weight loss journey, please drop by the ELH website http://easyleanandhealthy.com – I'm happy to help in any way I can.

Wishing you the best in health,

Robert Lalonde

ABOUT THE AUTHOR

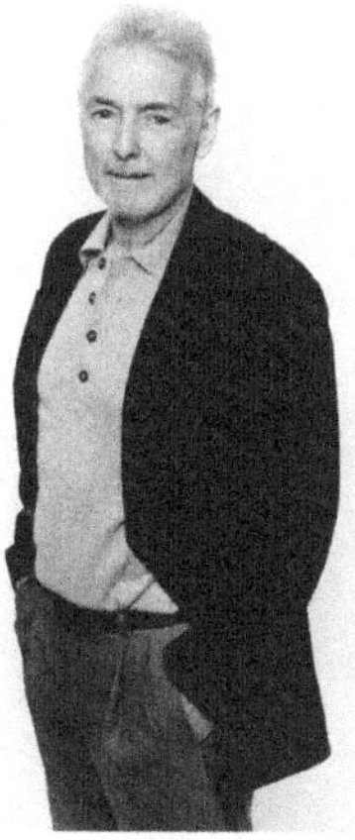

Robert Lalonde is the author of The ELH Diet – Permanent Weight Loss With A Healthy Diet Plan.

Robert studied Real Estate Appraisal in college and Real Property Assessment through UBC. He worked as a Commercial Property Tax Consultant in Toronto, Canada, representing owners of hotels, office buildings and shopping malls before various tribunals for tax appeals.

He is a recent cancer survivor living in the Georgian Bay area of Ontario, Canada with his wife Marianne and their Shi Tzu, Lucy.

INDEX

T

Made in the USA
Monee, IL
04 November 2026

67385524R00089